500
Rowing Machine
Workouts Book

500 Rowing Machine Workouts Book

Row to Fitness with 500 Dynamic Rowing Workouts for Ultimate Strength and Cardio Mastery

Logging Sheets (electronic format)
Are Available by a Scanning QR Code

Be.Bull Publishing Group

Toronto, Canada

500 Rowing Machine Workouts
Book by Be.Bull Publishing Group (Aria Capri International Inc.). All Rights Reserved.

Authors:

Be.Bull Publishing Group
Mauricio Vasquez

First Printing: April 2024

ISBN 978-1-998402-28-1 (Hardcover)
ISBN 978-1-998402-29-8 (Paperback)

FREE DOWNLOAD

BONUS No 1

Get the LOGGING SHEETS for free!

Just scan the QR code in this book. You can download them to your computer or laptop.

Print as many copies as you need to keep track of your workouts, or you can even fill them out on your device.

(QR code is found at the end of this book)

TIPS

- Adjust the intensity and duration of your rowing sessions according to your capabilities, skills, and physical condition. Personalization is key to effective training and preventing injuries.
- Listen to your body and don't push yourself too hard. Recognize the difference between challenging yourself and overtraining. Rest and recovery are just as important as the workouts themselves.
- Have your workout plan ready before you start. Knowing exactly what rowing intervals you're doing will make your workout more efficient and effective.
- Create a motivational playlist to keep you energized. Music can be a powerful motivator during rowing exercises, helping you to maintain pace and intensity.
- Minimize distractions by putting your phone on airplane mode during workouts. This helps you stay focused on your form, breathing, and the execution of each exercise.
- Incorporate dynamic stretching into your warm-up routine. Properly preparing your muscles and joints for rowing exercises reduces the risk of injury and enhances performance.
- Choose the appropriate difficulty level. Since there's no "weight" to adjust, modify exercises to match your fitness level.
- Keep a workout log to track your progress. Note the details of each rowing session and bodyweight exercise routine, including time, intensity, and repetitions, to see your improvement over time.
- Enjoy your workouts and the process of becoming fitter and stronger. Find joy in the challenges and celebrate your achievements, no matter how small they may seem.

These tips encourage a personalized, safe, and enjoyable approach to fitness, emphasizing the importance of listening to your body, preparing adequately, and staying motivated throughout the journey of rowing training.

Disclaimer

Be.Bull Publishing (Aria Capri International Inc.) strongly recommends that you consult with your physician before beginning any exercise program or workout. You should be in good physical condition and be able to participate in the exercises and workouts. We are not a licensed medical care provider and represents that we have no expertise in diagnosing, examining, or treating medical conditions of any kind, or in determining the effect of any specific exercise or workout on a medical condition.

You should understand that when participating in any exercise or workout, there is the possibility of physical injury. If you engage in the exercises and workouts of this book, you agree that you do so at your own risk, are voluntarily participating in these activities, assume all risk of injury to yourself, and agree to release and discharge Be.Bull Publishing (Aria Capri International Inc.) from any and all claims or causes of action, known or unknown, arising out of this book and videos.

The information provided through this book is not intended to be a substitute for professional medical advice, diagnosis or treatment. Never disregard professional medical advice, or delay in seeking it, because of something you have read on this book or watch in the videos. Never rely on information on this book or videos in place of seeking professional medical advice.

Be.Bull Publishing (Aria Capri International Inc.) is not responsible or liable for any advice, course of treatment, diagnosis or any other information, services or products that you obtain through this book or videos. You are encouraged to consult with your doctor with regard to the information contained on or through this book or videos. After reading this book or watching videos from this book, you are encouraged to review the information carefully with your professional healthcare provider.

If you want to add more variety to your workouts, scan this QR code to check these workout books!

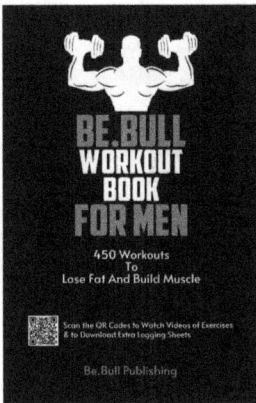

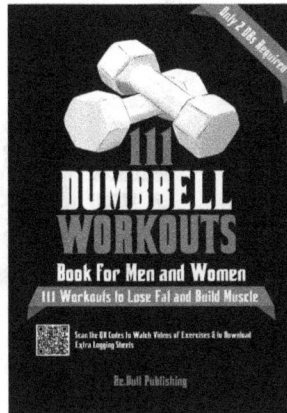

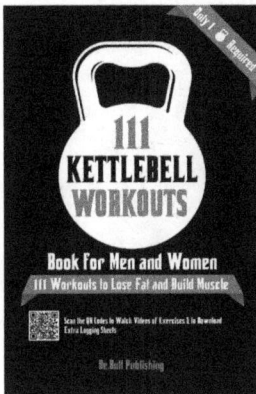

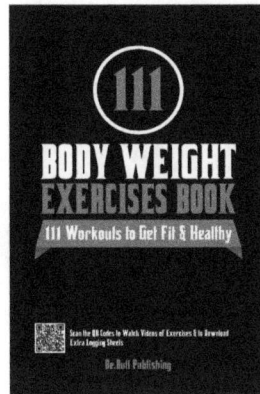

BE.BULL WORKOUT BOOK FOR MEN

450 Workouts To Lose Fat And Build Muscle

Scan the QR Codes to Watch Videos of Exercises & to Download Extra Logging Sheets

Be.Bull Publishing

111 DUMBBELL WORKOUTS

Book For Men and Women

111 Workouts to Lose Fat and Build Muscle

Only 2 DBs Required

Scan the QR Codes to Watch Videos of Exercises & to Download Extra Logging Sheets

Be.Bull Publishing

111 KETTLEBELL WORKOUTS

Book For Men and Women

111 Workouts to Lose Fat and Build Muscle

Only 1 KB Required

Scan the QR Codes to Watch Videos of Exercises & to Download Extra Logging Sheets

Be.Bull Publishing

111 BODY WEIGHT EXERCISES BOOK

111 Workouts to Get Fit & Healthy

Scan the QR Codes to Watch Videos of Exercises & to Download Extra Logging Sheets

Be.Bull Publishing

Dear valued customer,

We are a small family-owned business, and we'd like to please kindly ask you to leave us a review.

We don't have the same budget as big publishing companies, so your support would be really appreciated. Your feedback will mean a lot to us, and we thank you in advance!

Mauricio & Devon

Workout No.	Objective	Focus	Workout
1	Cardiovascular Endurance	Maintain a steady pace on the rower and focus on smooth transitions between exercises for efficiency.	(1) Row 500 meters
			Total Rounds: 4
			with a 2-minute rest between rounds.
2	Cardiovascular Endurance	Keep a consistent pace on the rower and maintain steady breathing throughout the workout.	(1) Row for 500 meters at a moderate pace
			Total Rounds: 4
			Time Cap: 20 minutes
3	Strength & Endurance	Focus on maintaining proper form during each exercise to maximize effectiveness.	(1) Row for 3 minutes at a high intensity
			Total Rounds: 3
			Rest 1 minute between rounds
4	Power & Speed	Explode powerfully on the rower and during the jump squats for maximum power output.	(1) Row for 1 minute at maximum effort
			Total Rounds: 5
			Rest 2 minutes between rounds
5	Agility & Coordination	Focus on quick transitions between exercises and maintaining balance during lunges.	(1) Row for 400 meters at a moderate pace
			Total Rounds: 4
			Time Cap: 25 minutes

Workout No.	Objective	Focus	Workout
6	High-Intensity Interval Training	Push yourself to the limit during the high-intensity intervals and focus on recovery.	(1) Row for 1 minute at sprint pace
			(4) 1 minute of rest
			Time Cap: 25 minutes
7	Core Strength	Engage your core during each exercise to improve stability and core strength.	(1) Row for 2 minutes at a moderate pace
			Total Rounds: 4
			Time Cap: 20 minutes
8	Endurance & Flexibility	Maintain a brisk pace on the rower and focus on stretching fully during the yoga poses.	(1) Row for 5 minutes at a steady pace
			Total Rounds: 3
			Time Cap: 30 minutes
9	Full Body Conditioning	Keep your movements controlled and deliberate to work every muscle group effectively.	(1) Row for 4 minutes at a moderate intensity
			Total Rounds: 3
			Time Cap: 25 minutes
10	Stamina & Resilience	Focus on pushing through fatigue and maintaining your pace on the rower and exercises.	(1) Row for 2 minutes at high intensity
			Total Rounds: 4
			Rest 2 minutes between rounds

Workout No.	Objective	Focus	Workout
11	Balance & Core Activation	Concentrate on engaging your core and maintaining balance during single-leg exercises.	(1) Row for 3 minutes at a steady pace
			Total Rounds: 4
			Time Cap: 25 minutes
12	Cardiovascular Endurance	Focus on consistent pace and rhythm; breathe deeply to maintain stamina.	(1) Row at a moderate intensity for 5,000 meters
			Time Cap: 25 minutes
13	High-Intensity Intervals	Push yourself to the max during sprints; rest fully during low intervals.	(1) 30 seconds of max effort rowing, followed by 30 seconds rest.
			Total Rounds: 20
			Total Time: 20 minutes
14	Steady-State Training	Maintain a constant, moderate pace, focusing on form and endurance.	(1) Row for 10,000 meters at a steady, moderate pace.
			Time Cap: 40 minutes
15	Speed and Recovery	Alternate between fast rowing and complete recovery to improve speed.	(1) 1 minute of sprint rowing, followed by 2 minutes of light rowing.
			Total Rounds: 10
			Total Time: 30 minutes
16	Aerobic Capacity	Keep a pace that challenges you but allows for conversation.	(1) Row for 60 minutes at a consistent, moderate intensity.
			Total Time: 60 minutes

Workout No.	Objective	Focus	Workout
17	Interval Pyramids	Increase intensity with each interval, then decrease in a pyramid pattern.	(1) Row for 1, 2, 3, 4, 3, 2, 1 minutes at high intensity, with 1 minute rest between.
			Total Time: 25 minutes
18	Threshold Training	Row at the highest pace you can sustain throughout the workout.	(1) Row for 2,000 meters as fast as possible
			Total Distance: 2,000 meters
19	Recovery Focus	Use rowing to actively recover, focusing on technique and relaxation.	(1) Row for 20 minutes at a light, easy pace.
			Total Time: 20 minutes
20	Endurance Building	Gradually increase rowing time to build endurance, focusing on persistence.	(1) Row for 30 minutes, increasing pace slightly every 10 minutes.
			Total Time: 30 minutes
21	Sprint Challenge	Test your power with short, maximum-effort sprints and ample recovery.	(1) 20 seconds of all-out sprint rowing, followed by 40 seconds of rest.
			Total Rounds: 12
			Total Time: 12 minutes
22	Full Body Conditioning	Keep your movements fluid and controlled, focusing on the transition between exercises.	(1) Row for 500 meters
			Total Rounds: 3
			Time Cap: 30 minutes

Workout No.	Objective	Focus	Workout
23	Cardiovascular & Strength Endurance	Maintain a steady pace on the rower and aim for consistent repetitions in each set.	(1) Row for 2 minutes at a high intensity
			Total Rounds: 4
			Time Cap: 40 minutes
24	Power & Speed	Focus on explosive movements for each exercise, aiming for maximum power and speed.	(1) Row for 1 minute at maximum effort
			Total Rounds: 5
			Rest 1 minute between rounds
25	HIIT & Agility	Move quickly between exercises with minimal rest, keeping your heart rate elevated.	(1) Row for 500 meters at a fast pace
			Total Rounds: 4
			Time Cap: 20 minutes
26	Core Stability & Endurance	Engage your core throughout the workout, focusing on stability during rowing and core exercises.	(1) Row for 3 minutes at moderate intensity
			Total Rounds: 3
			Time Cap: 25 minutes
27	Aerobic Capacity Building	Aim for a consistent aerobic effort that challenges you but is sustainable.	(1) Row for 4 minutes at a steady pace
			Total Rounds: 4
			Time Cap: 30 minutes

Workout No.	Objective	Focus	Workout
28	Interval Training	Alternate between high intensity on the rower and active recovery with bodyweight exercises.	(1) Row for 1 minute at high intensity
			Total Rounds: 6
			Time Cap: 24 minutes
30	Speed Endurance	Focus on maintaining speed during rowing and quick transitions to bodyweight exercises.	(1) Row for 3 minutes at high intensity
			Total Rounds: 3
			Time Cap: 25 minutes
31	Recovery & Technique	Use this session to focus on rowing technique and gentle bodyweight movement for recovery.	(1) Row for 5 minutes at a light pace
			Total Rounds: 2
			Time Cap: 20 minutes
32	Cardiovascular Endurance	Keep a consistent stroke rate, focusing on long, powerful pulls for efficiency.	(1) Row for 30 minutes at a moderate pace.
			Total Time: 30 minutes
33	High-Intensity Interval Training (HIIT)	Alternate between maximum effort and rest, focusing on quick recovery during low intervals.	(1) 1 minute of rowing at high intensity, followed by 1 minute of rest.
			Total Rounds: 10
			Total Time: 20 minutes

Workout No.	Objective	Focus	Workout
34	Speed Work	Concentrate on increasing your stroke rate while maintaining form for speed improvement.	(1) Row for 500 meters at max effort, then 3 minutes of rest
			Total Rounds: 5
			Total Distance: 2,500 meters
35	Aerobic Power	Maintain a steady but challenging pace, focusing on breathing and rhythm.	(1) Row for 2,000 meters at a steady pace.
			Total Time: Aim to complete as fast as possible
36	Recovery Rowing	Use this workout for active recovery, focusing on smooth, steady strokes.	(1) Row at a light pace for 20 minutes, concentrating on form.
			Total Time: 20 minutes
37	Threshold Training	Push to maintain a pace just below your sprint speed, focusing on endurance.	(1) Row for 4 minutes at high intensity, followed by 2 minutes of light rowing
			Total Rounds: 5
			Total Time: 30 minutes
38	Progressive Intervals	Gradually increase intensity with each interval, focusing on maintaining technique under fatigue.	(1) Row for 1 minute at moderate pace, 2 minutes at moderate-high, 3 minutes at high intensity, then reverse.
			Total Time: 12 minutes
39	Ladder Workout	Increase distance with each round, focusing on maintaining a consistent pace throughout.	(1) Row 250 meters, rest 1 minute, row 500 meters, rest 1 minute, up to 1,000 meters
			Total Time: Based on individual pace

Workout No.	Objective	Focus	Workout
40	Sprint Recovery Mix	Focus on all-out sprints followed by adequate recovery to enhance speed and recovery efficiency.	(1) 30 seconds of sprint rowing, followed by 1 minute of rest.
			Total Rounds: 15
			Total Time: 22.5 minutes
41	Endurance Challenge	Aim to keep a consistent pace for an extended period, focusing on mental and physical stamina.	(1) Row for 10,000 meters at a moderate, consistent pace.
			Total Distance: 10,000 meters
42	Cardio & Strength	Focus on maintaining high energy levels during rowing and precise form during bodyweight exercises.	(1) Row for 500 meters
			Total Rounds: 3
			Time Cap: 25 minutes
43	High-Intensity Interval Training	Alternate intense rowing bursts with active recovery bodyweight exercises to keep the heart rate up.	(1) Row for 1 minute at max effort
			Total Rounds: 6
			Time Cap: 20 minutes
44	Endurance & Core Stability	Balance prolonged rowing periods with exercises that enhance core stability and endurance.	(1) Row for 1,000 meters
			Total Rounds: 2
			Time Cap: 30 minutes

Workout No.	Objective	Focus	Workout
40	Sprint Recovery Mix	Focus on all-out sprints followed by adequate recovery to enhance speed and recovery efficiency.	(1) 30 seconds of sprint rowing, followed by 1 minute of rest.
			Total Rounds: 15
			Total Time: 22.5 minutes
41	Endurance Challenge	Aim to keep a consistent pace for an extended period, focusing on mental and physical stamina.	(1) Row for 10,000 meters at a moderate, consistent pace.
			Total Distance: 10,000 meters
42	Cardio & Strength	Focus on maintaining high energy levels during rowing and precise form during bodyweight exercises.	(1) Row for 500 meters
			Total Rounds: 3
			Time Cap: 25 minutes
43	High-Intensity Interval Training	Alternate intense rowing bursts with active recovery bodyweight exercises to keep the heart rate up.	(1) Row for 1 minute at max effort
			Total Rounds: 6
			Time Cap: 20 minutes
44	Endurance & Core Stability	Balance prolonged rowing periods with exercises that enhance core stability and endurance.	(1) Row for 1,000 meters
			Total Rounds: 2
			Time Cap: 30 minutes

Workout No.	Objective	Focus	Workout
45	Agility & Speed	Focus on quick transitions between rowing and bodyweight exercises to improve agility and speed.	(1) Row for 3 minutes at high intensity
			Total Rounds: 4
			Rest 1 minute between rounds
46	Power & Explosiveness	Concentrate on explosive power during both rowing sprints and plyometric exercises.	(1) Row for 500 meters at max effort
			Total Rounds: 3
			Time Cap: 25 minutes
47	Aerobic & Anaerobic Conditioning	Aim to push the limits of both your aerobic and anaerobic capacities.	(1) Row for 2 minutes at moderate intensity
			Total Rounds: 4
			Time Cap: 30 minutes
48	Recovery & Mobility	Use this workout as a recovery day, focusing on technique and stretching.	(1) Row for 5 minutes at a light pace
			Total Rounds: 3
			Time Cap: 30 minutes
49	Full Body Workout	Engage all major muscle groups with a combination of rowing and bodyweight exercises.	(1) Row for 4 minutes at steady pace
			Total Rounds: 3
			Time Cap: 35 minutes

Workout No.	Objective	Focus	Workout
50	Speed Endurance	Focus on maintaining speed on the rower and quick execution of bodyweight exercises.	(1) Row for 1 minute at high intensity
			Total Rounds: 5
			Time Cap: 25 minutes
51	Interval Challenge	Push for maximum effort during rowing intervals and maintain intensity with bodyweight exercises.	(1) Row for 2 minutes at max effort
			Total Rounds: 4
			Time Cap: 20 minutes
52	Aerobic Endurance	Focus on maintaining a consistent pace that allows for conversation throughout.	(1) Row for 30 minutes at a steady pace
			Total Time: 30 minutes
53	Anaerobic Threshold	Push yourself to maintain the highest pace you can sustain without slowing.	(1) Row for 8 minutes at high intensity, 2 minutes rest.
			Total Rounds: 3
			Total Time: 30 minutes
54	Interval Sprints	Concentrate on explosive starts and quick recovery during short rest periods.	(1) Row 250 meters at maximum effort, then rest for 1 minute.
			Total Rounds: 10
			Total Distance: 2,500 meters

Workout No.	Objective	Focus	Workout
55	Steady State Rowing	Keep a uniform stroke rate and focus on breathing and technique.	(1) Row for 45 minutes at a moderate, consistent pace.
			Total Time: 45 minutes
56	High-Intensity Intervals	Alternate between pushing hard on the rower and resting for short periods.	(1) 1 minute of rowing at maximum effort, followed by 1 minute of rest.
			Total Rounds: 15
			Total Time: 30 minutes
57	Recovery Row	Use this time to focus on technique, with light intensity for active recovery.	(1) Row for 20 minutes at a light pace
			Total Time: 20 minutes
58	Progressive Distance	Gradually increase the rowing distance each round to build endurance.	(1) Row 500 meters, then increase by 500 meters each round up to 2,000 meters
			Total Distance: 4,500 meters
59	Time Trial	Test your limits by rowing a set distance as fast as possible.	(1) Row 2,000 meters as fast as possible
			Total Distance: 2,000 meters
60	Pyramid Intervals	Increase and then decrease rowing time for varied intensity.	(1) Row for 1, 2, 3, 4, 3, 2, 1 minutes at high intensity with 1 minute of rest between intervals
			Total Time: 21 minutes (including rest)
61	Sprint Recovery	Focus on full-power sprints followed by equal time for recovery.	(1) 30 seconds of all-out sprinting, followed by 30 seconds of light rowing.
			Total Rounds: 20
			Total Time: 20 minutes

Workout No.	Objective	Focus	Workout
55	Steady State Rowing	Keep a uniform stroke rate and focus on breathing and technique.	(1) Row for 45 minutes at a moderate, consistent pace. Total Time: 45 minutes
56	High-Intensity Intervals	Alternate between pushing hard on the rower and resting for short periods.	(1) 1 minute of rowing at maximum effort, followed by 1 minute of rest. Total Rounds: 15 Total Time: 30 minutes
57	Recovery Row	Use this time to focus on technique, with light intensity for active recovery.	(1) Row for 20 minutes at a light pace Total Time: 20 minutes
58	Progressive Distance	Gradually increase the rowing distance each round to build endurance.	(1) Row 500 meters, then increase by 500 meters each round up to 2,000 meters Total Distance: 4,500 meters
59	Time Trial	Test your limits by rowing a set distance as fast as possible.	(1) Row 2,000 meters as fast as possible Total Distance: 2,000 meters
60	Pyramid Intervals	Increase and then decrease rowing time for varied intensity.	(1) Row for 1, 2, 3, 4, 3, 2, 1 minutes at high intensity with 1 minute of rest between intervals Total Time: 21 minutes (including rest)
61	Sprint Recovery	Focus on full-power sprints followed by equal time for recovery.	(1) 30 seconds of all-out sprinting, followed by 30 seconds of light rowing. Total Rounds: 20 Total Time: 20 minutes

Workout No.	Objective	Focus	Workout
67	Agility & Speed	Focus on quick transitions between rowing and bodyweight exercises to improve agility.	(1) Row for 2 minutes at high intensity
			Total Rounds: 5
			Rest 1 minute between rounds
68	Progressive Overload	Gradually increase the rowing distance each round to build up endurance and strength.	(1) Row for 250 meters
			Increase rowing by 250 meters each round
			Total Rounds: 4
			Final Row: 1,000 meters
69	Recovery & Technique	Use this workout for active recovery, focusing on rowing technique and light bodyweight movement.	(1) Row at a light pace for 5 minutes
			Total Rounds: 3
			Time Cap: 30 minutes
70	Speed Endurance	Combine fast-paced rowing with endurance bodyweight exercises for a challenging workout.	(1) Row for 1 minute at maximum effort
			Total Rounds: 6
			Time Cap: 25 minutes
71	Interval Challenge	Push for maximum effort during rowing intervals and maintain intensity with quick bodyweight exercises.	(1) Row for 2 minutes at max effort
			Total Rounds: 4

Workout No.	Objective	Focus	Workout
73	High-Intensity Intervals	Push to your limit during the high-intensity periods and focus on recovering during the rest periods.	(1) 30 seconds of rowing at maximum effort, followed by 30 seconds of rest.
			Total Rounds: 20
			Total Time: 20 minutes
74	Steady-State Endurance	Aim for a steady pace that challenges you but is sustainable for the entire duration.	(1) Row for 45 minutes at a consistent pace.
			Total Time: 45 minutes
75	Sprint Training	Concentrate on explosive power from the start of each sprint, aiming for maximum speed.	(1) 1 minute of rowing at sprint pace, then 2 minutes of rest.
			Total Rounds: 10
			Total Time: 30 minutes
76	Threshold Workout	Work at or near your anaerobic threshold to improve your ability to sustain high-intensity efforts.	(1) Row for 5 minutes at high intensity, then 5 minutes at a recovery pace.
			Total Rounds: 4
			Total Time: 40 minutes
77	Recovery Row	Focus on technique and use this time for active recovery, maintaining a low intensity.	(1) Row at a light pace for 30 minutes.
			Total Time: 30 minutes
78	Interval Pyramids	Build intensity with each interval before reducing the effort in a pyramid fashion.	(1) Row for 1, 2, 3, 4, 3, 2, 1 minutes at high intensity with 1 minute of rest between each.
			Total Time: 27 minutes
79	Time Trial	Test your performance over a set distance, focusing on maintaining a fast, consistent pace.	(1) Row 2,000 meters as fast as possible
			Total Distance: 2,000 meters

Workout No.	Objective	Focus	Workout
80	Variable Intensity	Alternate between different intensity levels to challenge your body's response to changing demands.	(1) Row for 3 minutes at high intensity, 2 minutes at moderate intensity, and 1 minute at easy pace.
			Total Rounds: 5
			Total Time: 30 minutes
81	Endurance and Technique	Focus on maintaining proper rowing technique over a longer duration for endurance building.	(1) Row for 60 minutes, focusing on technique and maintaining a consistent stroke rate
			Total Time: 60 minutes
82	Full Body Conditioning	Concentrate on smooth transitions between rowing and bodyweight exercises to maintain intensity.	(1) Row for 500 meters
			Total Rounds: 4
			Time Cap: 30 minutes
83	Cardio & Strength Endurance	Maintain a steady pace on the rower and focus on form for bodyweight exercises.	(1) Row for 3 minutes at moderate intensity
			Total Rounds: 3
			Time Cap: 25 minutes
84	HIIT & Core Stability	Push hard during rowing intervals and engage your core during bodyweight exercises.	(1) Row for 1 minute at high intensity
			Total Rounds: 6
			Time Cap: 20 minutes
85	Endurance & Flexibility	Aim for long rowing sessions with stretching exercises in between to improve flexibility.	(1) Row for 1000 meters
			Total Rounds: 3
			Time Cap: 35 minutes

Workout No.	Objective	Focus	Workout
86	Power & Agility	Focus on explosive power during rowing sprints and agility in bodyweight movements.	(1) Row for 250 meters at sprint pace
			Total Rounds: 5
			Time Cap: 30 minutes
87	Speed & Coordination	Enhance your coordination with fast-paced rowing and quick bodyweight exercises.	(1) Row for 2 minutes at high intensity
			Total Rounds: 4
			Rest 1 minute between rounds
88	Aerobic Capacity & Strength	Build aerobic capacity on the rower and strength through bodyweight resistance.	(1) Row for 5 minutes at steady state
			Total Rounds: 3
			Time Cap: 30 minutes
89	Recovery & Mobility	Use rowing for active recovery and bodyweight exercises to enhance mobility.	(1) Row at a light pace for 5 minutes
			Total Rounds: 2
			Time Cap: 20 minutes
90	Interval Challenge	Integrate high-intensity rowing with challenging bodyweight circuits for a comprehensive workout.	(1) Row for 1 minute at max effort
			Total Rounds: 5
			Time Cap: 25 minutes
91	Endurance & Technique Focus	Focus on rowing technique for efficiency and bodyweight exercises for functional strength.	(1) Row for 6 minutes focusing on technique
			Total Rounds: 4
			Time Cap: 40 minutes

Workout No.	Objective	Focus	Workout
92	Aerobic Base Building	Keep a steady pace that you can maintain for the entire duration to build your aerobic base.	(1) Row for 60 minutes at a moderate pace
			Total Time: 60 minutes
93	High-Intensity Intervals	Focus on maximum effort during sprints and complete recovery during rests to improve power and speed.	(1) 1 minute of rowing at maximum effort, followed by 1 minute of rest.
			Total Rounds: 20
			Total Time: 40 minutes
94	Steady-State Endurance	Maintain a constant, challenging pace that tests your endurance without overexerting.	(1) Row for 30 minutes at a steady pace.
			Total Time: 30 minutes
95	Sprint Training	Concentrate on explosive power and quick starts during each sprint to increase your speed.	(1) 30 seconds of all-out sprinting, followed by 2 minutes of easy rowing.
			Total Rounds: 10
			Total Time: 25 minutes
96	Threshold Work	Aim to row at your anaerobic threshold, balancing on the edge of aerobic and anaerobic work.	(1) Row for 5 minutes at high intensity, then 5 minutes at a low intensity.
			Total Rounds: 4
			Total Time: 40 minutes
97	Recovery Row	Use this workout to focus on form and recovery, rowing at a low intensity.	(1) Row at a light pace for 20 minutes.
			Total Time: 20 minutes
98	Interval Pyramids	Increase and then decrease the length of your efforts in a pyramid format to challenge endurance and recovery.	(1) Row for 1, 2, 3, 4, 3, 2, 1 minutes at high intensity, with equal rest.
			Total Time: 28 minutes

Workout No.	Objective	Focus	Workout
99	Time Trial	Test your speed and endurance by rowing a set distance as fast as possible.	(1) Row 2,000 meters as fast as possible.
			Total Distance: 2,000 meters
100	Variable Intensity	Alternate between different intensity levels within the same workout to simulate race conditions or varied terrain.	(1) Row for 4 minutes at high intensity, 1 minute at low intensity.
			Total Rounds: 6
			Total Time: 30 minutes
101	Endurance and Technique Focus	Focus on maintaining efficient technique while building endurance over a long, steady row.	(1) Row for 75 minutes, concentrating on maintaining proper form throughout
			Total Time: 75 minutes
102	Comprehensive Fitness	Balance your effort between rowing and bodyweight exercises for full-body conditioning.	(1) Row for 4 minutes at moderate intensity
			Total Rounds: 4
			Time Cap: 30 minutes
103	Endurance & Core Strength	Keep a consistent pace on the rower and concentrate on engaging your core during bodyweight exercises.	(1) Row for 5 minutes
			Total Rounds: 3
			Time Cap: 30 minutes
104	High-Intensity Interval Training	Push hard on the rower for short bursts and maintain intensity with quick bodyweight movements.	(1) Row for 1 minute at high intensity
			Total Rounds: 7
			Time Cap: 20 minutes

Workout No.	Objective	Focus	Workout
105	Power & Speed	Focus on explosive power during rowing and fast-paced, powerful bodyweight exercises.	(1) Row for 500 meters at max effort
			Total Rounds: 4
			Time Cap: 25 minutes
106	Cardiovascular Endurance	Aim for longer, steady-state rowing intervals with endurance-based bodyweight exercises.	(1) Row for 10 minutes at a steady pace
			Total Rounds: 2
			Time Cap: 30 minutes
107	Agility & Coordination	Use rowing to improve cardiovascular fitness and bodyweight exercises to enhance agility and coordination.	(1) Row for 2 minutes at high intensity
			Total Rounds: 5
			Time Cap: 25 minutes
108	Recovery & Flexibility	Focus on low-intensity rowing and bodyweight exercises that promote flexibility and recovery.	(1) Row for 5 minutes at a light pace
			Total Rounds: 2
			Time Cap: 30 minutes
109	Anaerobic Threshold	Challenge your anaerobic capacity with intense rowing intervals and strength-building bodyweight exercises.	(1) Row for 2 minutes at max effort
			Total Rounds: 4
			Time Cap: 30 minutes
110	Interval Challenge	Alternate between rowing and bodyweight exercises for a challenging interval workout.	(1) Row for 3 minutes at high intensity
			Total Rounds: 5
			Time Cap: 30 minutes

Workout No.	Objective	Focus	Workout
111	Endurance & Technique	Maintain proper technique on the rower and during bodyweight exercises for efficient, injury-free workouts.	(1) Row for 6 minutes focusing on form
			Total Rounds: 4
			Time Cap: 40 minutes
112	Cardiovascular Endurance	Focus on maintaining a consistent pace, aiming for steady strokes and controlled breathing.	(1) Row for 30 minutes at a moderate, steady pace
			Total Time: 30 minutes
113	High-Intensity Intervals	Push yourself to the limit during high-intensity periods and focus on recovery during rest periods.	(1) 1 minute of rowing at maximum effort, followed by 1 minute of rest
			Total Rounds: 15
			Total Time: 30 minutes
114	Speed Work	Concentrate on increasing your stroke rate for speed improvement while maintaining good form.	(1) Row for 500 meters at max effort, followed by 2 minutes of rest.
			Total Rounds: 5
			Total Distance: 2,500 meters
115	Aerobic Power	Maintain a steady but challenging pace that allows you to work just below your maximum capacity.	(1) Row for 2,000 meters at a challenging pace.
			Total Time: Aim to complete as fast as possible
116	Recovery Rowing	Use this workout for active recovery, focusing on technique and keeping the intensity low.	(1) Row at a light pace for 20 minutes
			Total Time: 20 minutes
117	Threshold Training	Aim to row at or near your anaerobic threshold, balancing on the edge of comfort.	(1) Row for 4 minutes at high intensity, followed by 2 minutes of easy rowing.
			Total Rounds: 6
			Total Time: 36 minutes

Workout No.	Objective	Focus	Workout
118	Interval Pyramids	Increase and then decrease rowing time for varied intensity, focusing on endurance and speed.	(1) Row for 1, 2, 3, 4, 3, 2, 1 minutes at high intensity with equal rest
			Total Time: 28 minutes
119	Time Trial	Test your limits by rowing a set distance as fast as possible, maintaining a high and consistent pace.	(1) Row 2,000 meters as fast as possible.
			Total Distance: 2,000 meters
120	Variable Intensity	Alternate between different intensity levels to simulate race conditions or varied terrain.	(1) Row for 3 minutes at high intensity, 2 minutes at moderate, 1 minute at easy pace. Repeat.
			Total Rounds: 4
			Total Time: 24 minutes
121	Endurance Challenge	Aim for long-duration rowing at a moderate pace, focusing on stamina and mental toughness.	(1) Row for 60 minutes, focusing on maintaining a consistent pace throughout.
			Total Time: 60 minutes
122	Full Body Conditioning	Balance your effort between rowing and bodyweight exercises for a comprehensive workout.	(1) Row for 500 meters
			Total Rounds: 3
			Time Cap: 30 minutes
123	High-Intensity Fat Burn	Push hard during rowing intervals and move quickly through bodyweight exercises to maximize calorie burn.	(1) Row for 1 minute at high intensity
			Total Rounds: 6
			Time Cap: 25 minutes
124	Endurance & Strength	Maintain a consistent pace on the rower and focus on maintaining proper form during bodyweight exercises.	(1) Row for 1000 meters
			Total Rounds: 4
			Time Cap: 40 minutes

Workout No.	Objective	Focus	Workout
125	Aerobic Capacity & Core	Keep your heart rate up with rowing and focus on core strength with bodyweight exercises.	(1) Row for 3 minutes at moderate intensity
			Total Rounds: 5
			Time Cap: 30 minutes
126	Cardio & Lower Body Strength	Focus on cardiovascular fitness with rowing and lower body strength with squats and lunges.	(1) Row for 4 minutes
			Total Rounds: 3
			Time Cap: 30 minutes
127	High-Intensity Interval Training (HIIT)	Alternate between intense rowing sessions and high-effort bodyweight exercises for a HIIT workout.	(1) Row for 1 minute at high intensity
			Total Rounds: 7
			Time Cap: 20 minutes
128	Recovery & Flexibility	Use rowing for light cardio and bodyweight exercises to promote flexibility and recovery.	(1) Row at a light pace for 5 minutes
			Total Rounds: 3
			Time Cap: 30 minutes
129	Speed & Coordination	Enhance your speed on the rower and coordination with dynamic bodyweight exercises.	(1) Row for 500 meters at high intensity
			Total Rounds: 5
			Time Cap: 25 minutes
130	Endurance & Technique	Concentrate on rowing technique for efficiency and bodyweight exercises for endurance.	(1) Row for 6 minutes focusing on form
			Total Rounds: 4
			Time Cap: 40 minutes

Workout No.	Objective	Focus	Workout
131	Cardiovascular Endurance	Maintain a consistent stroke rate and focus on efficient breathing throughout the workout.	(1) Row for 45 minutes at a moderate intensity.
			Total Time: 45 minutes
132	High-Intensity Interval Training	Push yourself to the limit during intense intervals and focus on recovery during rest periods.	(1) 2 minutes of rowing at high intensity, followed by 1 minute of rest
			Total Rounds: 10
			Total Time: 30 minutes
133	Steady-State Rowing	Aim for a steady pace that you can maintain for a long duration, focusing on endurance.	(1) Row for 60 minutes at a consistent, moderate pace
			Total Time: 60 minutes
134	Speed Work	Focus on increasing your stroke rate for short bursts to improve overall rowing speed.	(1) 30 seconds of sprint rowing, followed by 2 minutes of easy rowing
			Total Rounds: 8
			Total Time: 20 minutes
135	Aerobic Capacity	Keep a moderate intensity that allows you to work on your aerobic fitness without overexerting.	(1) Row for 20 minutes at a steady pace
			Total Time: 20 minutes
136	Threshold Training	Push to row at your anaerobic threshold, improving your ability to sustain high-intensity efforts.	(1) Row for 5 minutes at high intensity, followed by 3 minutes of rest.
			Total Rounds: 5
			Total Time: 40 minutes
137	Recovery Row	Use this session for active recovery, focusing on light intensity and proper technique.	(1) Row at a light pace for 30 minutes, concentrating on form
			Total Time: 30 minutes

Workout No.	Objective	Focus	Workout
138	Interval Pyramids	Build up the intensity with each interval before decreasing, focusing on endurance and speed.	(1) Row for 1, 2, 3, 4, 3, 2, 1 minutes at high intensity, with 1 minute rest in between.
			Total Time: 25 minutes
139	Time Trial	Test your limits with a distance challenge, focusing on consistent power and pacing.	(1) Row 2000 meters as fast as possible.
			Total Distance: 2000 meters
140	Variable Intensity Training	Alternate between various intensity levels within the workout to challenge your body's response to changing demands.	(1) Row for 3 minutes at high intensity, 2 minutes at moderate, and 1 minute at easy pace. Repeat 3 times.
			Total Time: 18 minutes
141	Total Body Conditioning	Keep your movements fluid between the rower and bodyweight exercises, focusing on engaging all muscle groups.	(1) Row for 500 meters
			Total Rounds: 3
			Time Cap: 30 minutes
142	High-Intensity Fat Burn	Push hard during the rowing intervals and move quickly through bodyweight exercises to keep your heart rate elevated.	(1) Row for 1 minute at high intensity
			Total Rounds: 6
			Time Cap: 25 minutes
143	Endurance & Core Strength	Maintain a consistent pace on the rower and concentrate on core engagement during bodyweight exercises.	(1) Row for 1000 meters
			Total Rounds: 4
			Time Cap: 40 minutes
144	Power & Agility	Aim for powerful strokes on the rower and quick, agile movements during bodyweight exercises.	(1) Row for 2 minutes at max effort
			Total Rounds: 4
			Time Cap: 25 minutes

Workout No.	Objective	Focus	Workout
145	Cardiovascular Endurance	Keep your heart rate up with consistent rowing intervals and focus on endurance during bodyweight exercises.	(1) Row for 4 minutes
			Total Rounds: 3
			Time Cap: 30 minutes
146	High-Intensity Interval Training	Alternate between intense rowing sessions and high-effort bodyweight exercises for a full HIIT workout.	(1) Row for 1 minute at high intensity
			Total Rounds: 7
			Time Cap: 20 minutes
147	Recovery & Flexibility	Use light rowing intervals for active recovery and include bodyweight exercises to promote flexibility and muscle recovery.	(1) Row at a light pace for 5 minutes
			Total Rounds: 3
			Time Cap: 30 minutes
148	Speed & Coordination	Enhance your coordination with fast-paced rowing and bodyweight exercises that require balance and precision.	(1) Row for 500 meters at high intensity
			Total Rounds: 5
			Time Cap: 25 minutes
149	Endurance & Technique	Focus on maintaining good rowing technique for efficiency and perform bodyweight exercises that enhance endurance and strength.	(1) Row for 6 minutes focusing on form
			Total Rounds: 4
			Time Cap: 40 minutes
150	Interval Challenge	Integrate challenging rowing intervals with bodyweight exercises designed to test your limits and improve your overall fitness.	(1) Row for 3 minutes at high intensity
			Total Rounds: 5
			Time Cap: 30 minutes

Workout No.	Objective	Focus	Workout
151	Cardiovascular Endurance	Focus on maintaining a steady pace, emphasizing endurance over speed.	(1) Row for 60 minutes at a moderate pace
			Total Time: 60 minutes
152	High-Intensity Intervals	Alternate between full effort and active recovery to boost cardiovascular and muscular endurance.	(1) 30 seconds of rowing at maximum effort, followed by 1 minute of light rowing.
			Total Rounds: 20
			Total Time: 30 minutes
153	Speed Work	Aim to increase your stroke rate while maintaining form, focusing on quick, powerful pulls.	(1) Row for 500 meters at maximum speed, then rest for 2 minutes.
			Total Rounds: 5
			Total Distance: 2,500 meters
154	Aerobic Capacity	Keep a moderate intensity to build aerobic base without overexerting.	(1) Row for 45 minutes at a consistent, moderate intensity.
			Total Time: 45 minutes
155	Recovery Rowing	Use this session for active recovery, focusing on technique and maintaining a low intensity.	(1) Row at a light pace for 30 minutes
			Total Time: 30 minutes
156	Threshold Training	Row at or near your anaerobic threshold to improve your ability to sustain high-intensity efforts longer.	(1) Row for 8 minutes at high intensity, followed by 2 minutes of rest.
			Total Rounds: 4
			Total Time: 40 minutes

Workout No.	Objective	Focus	Workout
157	Interval Pyramids	Build endurance and speed with pyramid intervals, increasing and then decreasing the effort.	(1) Row for 1, 2, 3, 4, 3, 2, 1 minutes at high intensity, with 1 minute of rest between intervals
			Total Time: 28 minutes
158	Time Trial	Challenge yourself to row a set distance as quickly as possible, focusing on consistent power output.	(1) Row 2000 meters as fast as possible.
			Total Distance: 2000 meters
159	Variable Intensity Training	Improve adaptability by varying intensity levels, simulating race conditions or different terrains.	(1) Row for 5 minutes at high intensity, 3 minutes at medium, and 2 minutes at easy pace. Repeat 2 times
			Total Time: 20 minutes
160	Endurance Challenge	Test your stamina with a long-distance row, focusing on maintaining a consistent pace throughout.	(1) Row for 10,000 meters at a steady pace.
			Total Distance: 10,000 meters
161	Full Body Conditioning	Engage your entire body by balancing effort between rowing and dynamic bodyweight exercises.	(1) Row for 500 meters
			Total Rounds: 3
			Time Cap: 30 minutes
162	Cardiovascular & Muscular Endurance	Maintain a consistent pace on the rower and focus on proper form for bodyweight exercises.	(1) Row for 3 minutes at moderate intensity
			Total Rounds: 4
			Time Cap: 40 minutes

Workout No.	Objective	Focus	Workout
163	High-Intensity Fat Burn	Alternate between high-intensity rowing and quick bodyweight movements to keep the heart rate elevated.	(1) Row for 1 minute at high intensity
			Total Rounds: 6
			Time Cap: 20 minutes
164	Strength & Power	Focus on explosive movements during rowing and plyometric bodyweight exercises.	(1) Row for 500 meters at max effort
			Total Rounds: 4
			Time Cap: 30 minutes
165	Agility & Coordination	Improve coordination and agility with fast-paced rowing and functional bodyweight movements.	(1) Row for 2 minutes at high intensity
			Total Rounds: 5
			Time Cap: 25 minutes
166	Recovery & Mobility	Use rowing for active recovery and include bodyweight exercises to enhance mobility.	(1) Row at a light pace for 5 minutes
			Total Rounds: 3
			Time Cap: 30 minutes
167	Aerobic & Anaerobic Conditioning	Challenge both your aerobic and anaerobic systems with varied intensity rowing and bodyweight exercises.	(1) Row for 4 minutes at moderate intensity
			Total Rounds: 4
			Time Cap: 30 minutes

Workout No.	Objective	Focus	Workout
168	Core Strength & Stability	Strengthen your core with a mix of rowing and targeted bodyweight exercises.	(1) Row for 3 minutes at steady state
			Total Rounds: 4
			Time Cap: 30 minutes
169	Endurance & Technique Focus	Aim for long-duration rowing intervals with technical bodyweight movements to improve endurance and form.	(1) Row for 6 minutes focusing on stroke consistency
			Total Rounds: 3
			Time Cap: 30 minutes
170	Interval Challenge	Integrate challenging rowing intervals with bodyweight exercises for a comprehensive high-intensity workout.	(1) Row for 2 minutes at max effort
			Total Rounds: 5
			Time Cap: 30 minutes
171	Aerobic Base Building	Maintain a consistent, moderate intensity to enhance cardiovascular endurance and aerobic capacity.	(1) Row for 60 minutes at a steady pace.
			Total Time: 60 minutes
172	High-Intensity Intervals	Maximize effort during sprints and fully recover during rest intervals to boost both aerobic and anaerobic fitness.	(1) 40 seconds of rowing at maximum effort, followed by 20 seconds of rest
			Total Rounds: 20
			Total Time: 20 minutes

Workout No.	Objective	Focus	Workout
173	Steady-State Endurance	Aim for a continuous, moderate effort, focusing on endurance and maintaining a consistent stroke	(1) Row for 45 minutes at a constant pace.
			Total Time: 45 minutes
174	Sprint Training	Focus on explosive starts and maintaining high speed for short distances to improve power and speed.	(1) 250 meters of rowing at sprint pace, then rest for 1 minute.
			Total Rounds: 8
			Total Distance: 2,000 meters
175	Threshold Work	Push to maintain a challenging pace just below your sprint level to increase your lactate threshold.	(1) Row for 4 minutes at high intensity, followed by 2 minutes of light rowing
			Total Rounds: 6
			Total Time: 36 minutes
176	Recovery Row	Use this workout to focus on rowing technique and recovery, keeping the intensity low and strokes smooth.	(1) Row at a light pace for 30 minutes.
			Total Time: 30 minutes
177	Interval Pyramids	Increase and then decrease the duration of your efforts in a pyramid format, challenging both endurance and speed.	(1) Row for 1, 2, 3, 4, 3, 2, 1 minutes at high intensity, with 1 minute of rest between intervals
			Total Time: 25 minutes
178	Time Trial	Challenge yourself with a distance-based test, focusing on pacing and maintaining a consistent effort throughout.	(1) Row 2000 meters as fast as possible
			Total Distance: 2000 meters

Workout No.	Objective	Focus	Workout
179	Variable Intensity	Simulate race conditions or varied terrain with changing intensities, focusing on adaptability and resilience.	(1) Row for 3 minutes at high intensity, 2 minutes at medium, and 1 minute at easy pace. Repeat 3 times.
			Total Time: 18 minutes
180	Endurance Challenge	Test your stamina with a long-distance row, focusing on maintaining a steady pace and efficient technique.	(1) Row for 10,000 meters at a steady, moderate pace
			Total Distance: 10,000 meters
181	Cardio & Strength Balance	Evenly distribute your effort between rowing for cardio and bodyweight exercises for strength.	(1) Row for 500 meters
			Total Rounds: 3
			Time Cap: 30 minutes
182	High-Intensity Fat Burn	Alternate intense rowing bursts with quick, high-intensity bodyweight exercises to maximize calorie burn.	(1) Row for 1 minute at high intensity
			Total Rounds: 6
			Time Cap: 20 minutes
183	Endurance & Core Strength	Maintain a steady pace on the rower; focus on core engagement during bodyweight exercises.	(1) Row for 1000 meters
			Total Rounds: 4
			Time Cap: 40 minutes
184	Power & Plyometrics	Focus on explosive power during rowing sprints and plyometric bodyweight exercises.	(1) Row for 500 meters at max effort
			Total Rounds: 4
			Time Cap: 30 minutes

Workout No.	Objective	Focus	Workout
185	Cardiovascular Endurance	Keep your heart rate up with consistent rowing intervals; focus on endurance during bodyweight exercises.	(1) Row for 4 minutes
			Total Rounds: 3
			Time Cap: 30 minutes
186	High-Intensity Interval Training	Alternate between intense rowing sessions and high-effort bodyweight exercises for a comprehensive HIIT workout.	(1) Row for 1 minute at high intensity
			Total Rounds: 7
			Time Cap: 20 minutes
187	Recovery & Mobility	Use rowing for active recovery and bodyweight exercises to promote flexibility and muscle recovery.	(1) Row at a light pace for 5 minutes
			Total Rounds: 3
			Time Cap: 30 minutes
188	Speed & Coordination	Enhance speed on the rower and coordination with dynamic bodyweight exercises.	(1) Row for 500 meters at high intensity
			Total Rounds: 5
			Time Cap: 25 minutes
189	Endurance & Technique	Focus on maintaining good rowing technique and endurance during longer bodyweight exercise sets.	(1) Row for 6 minutes focusing on form
			Total Rounds: 4
			Time Cap: 40 minutes

Workout No.	Objective	Focus	Workout
190	Interval Challenge	Integrate challenging rowing intervals with bodyweight exercises to test limits and improve overall fitness.	(1) Row for 2 minutes at max effort
			Total Rounds: 5
			Time Cap: 30 minutes
192	High-Intensity Intervals	Push your limits during high-intensity intervals and focus on quick recovery during rest periods.	(1) 1 minute of rowing at maximum effort, followed by 1 minute of rest.
			Total Rounds: 15
			Total Time: 30 minutes
193	Aerobic Capacity	Maintain a moderate intensity that challenges your aerobic system without overwhelming it.	(1) Row for 45 minutes at a steady, moderate intensity.
			Total Time: 45 minutes
194	Sprint Training	Concentrate on explosive power during sprints to increase your speed and power.	(1) 30 seconds of all-out sprinting, followed by 1 minute of easy rowing
			Total Rounds: 10
			Total Time: 20 minutes
195	Threshold Training	Work at or just below your anaerobic threshold to increase your ability to sustain high-intensity efforts.	(1) Row for 5 minutes at high intensity, followed by 3 minutes of easy rowing
			Total Rounds: 5
			Total Time: 40 minutes

Workout No.	Objective	Focus	Workout
196	Interval Pyramids	Build endurance and power with pyramid intervals, gradually increasing and then decreasing the effort.	(1) Row for 1, 2, 3, 4, 3, 2, 1 minutes at high intensity, with 1 minute of rest between each.
			Total Time: 28 minutes
197	Time Trial	Test your performance and stamina by rowing a set distance as quickly as possible.	(1) Row 2000 meters as fast as possible.
			Total Distance: 2000 meters
198	Variable Intensity Training	Improve adaptability by varying intensity levels, simulating race conditions or varied terrains.	(1) Row for 2 minutes at high intensity, 2 minutes at moderate, 1 minute at low intensity. Repeat 4 times.
			Total Time: 20 minutes
199	Endurance and Technique	Focus on long-duration rowing while maintaining efficient technique for stamina and performance improvement.	(1) Row for 60 minutes, concentrating on maintaining proper form and consistent stroke rate
			Total Time: 60 minutes
200	Total Body Conditioning	Balance effort between rowing for cardio and bodyweight exercises for strength and agility.	(1) Row for 500 meters
			Total Rounds: 3
			Time Cap: 30 minutes
201	Cardiovascular & Muscular Endurance	Maintain a consistent pace on the rower; focus on form and endurance during bodyweight exercises.	(1) Row for 3 minutes at moderate intensity
			Total Rounds: 4
			Time Cap: 40 minutes

Workout No.	Objective	Focus	Workout
202	High-Intensity Fat Burn	Push hard during rowing intervals; quickly transition to bodyweight exercises to keep heart rate elevated.	(1) Row for 1 minute at high intensity
			Total Rounds: 6
			Time Cap: 20 minutes
203	Cardiovascular Endurance	Keep heart rate up with consistent rowing intervals; include endurance bodyweight exercises.	(1) Row for 5 minutes
			Total Rounds: 3
			Time Cap: 35 minutes
204	Recovery & Mobility	Use rowing for active recovery and bodyweight exercises to enhance mobility and flexibility.	(1) Row at a light pace for 5 minutes
			(2) 5 minutes of Dynamic Stretching focusing on major muscle groups
			Total Rounds: 3
			Time Cap: 30 minutes
205	Endurance & Technique	Focus on rowing technique for efficiency and endurance during longer bodyweight exercise sets.	(1) Row for 6 minutes focusing on form
			Total Rounds: 4
			Time Cap: 40 minutes
206	Interval Challenge	Integrate challenging rowing intervals with bodyweight exercises for a full-body workout.	(1) Row for 2 minutes at max effort
			Total Rounds: 5
			Time Cap: 30 minutes

Workout No.	Objective	Focus	Workout
207	Aerobic Endurance	Maintain a consistent pace, focusing on long, powerful strokes for efficiency.	(1) Row for 45 minutes at a moderate pace.
			Total Time: 45 minutes
208	High-Intensity Intervals	Push to your limit during sprints and focus on quick recovery during rest periods.	(1) 1 minute of rowing at maximum effort, followed by 1 minute of rest.
			Total Rounds: 20
			Total Time: 40 minutes
209	Speed Work	Concentrate on increasing your stroke rate for short bursts to improve overall rowing speed.	(1) 500 meters of sprint rowing, then 2 minutes of rest.
			Total Rounds: 8
			Total Distance: 4,000 meters
210	Aerobic Capacity	Keep a moderate intensity to build your aerobic base without overexerting.	(1) Row for 20 minutes at a steady pace
			Total Time: 20 minutes
211	Recovery Row	Use this session for active recovery, focusing on technique and keeping the intensity low.	(1) Row at a light pace for 30 minutes
			Total Time: 30 minutes
212	Threshold Training	Work at or just below your anaerobic threshold to improve your ability to sustain high-intensity efforts.	(1) Row for 7 minutes at high intensity, followed by 3 minutes of easy rowing.
			Total Rounds: 5Total Time: 50 minutes
213	Interval Pyramids	Build endurance and speed with pyramid intervals, gradually increasing and then decreasing the effort.	(1) Row for 1, 2, 3, 4, 3, 2, 1 minutes at high intensity, with 1 minute of rest between each.
			Total Time: 27 minutes

Workout No.	Objective	Focus	Workout
214	Variable Intensity	Improve adaptability by varying intensity levels within the workout to simulate race conditions.	(1) Row for 3 minutes at high intensity, 2 minutes at moderate, 1 minute at easy pace. Repeat 4 times.
			Total Time: 24 minutes
215	Endurance Challenge	Test your stamina with a long-distance row, focusing on maintaining a steady pace throughout.	(1) Row for 10,000 meters at a steady, moderate pace
			Total Distance: 10,000 meters
216	Progressive Intervals	Gradually increase rowing time each round to build endurance and strength.	(1) Row for 2, 4, 6, 8, 6, 4, 2 minutes with 2 minutes rest between intervals
			Total Time: 42 minutes
217	Technique & Efficiency	Focus on refining rowing technique for efficiency, targeting stroke length and consistency.	(1) Row for 3 sets of 15 minutes focusing on technique, 5 minutes rest between sets
			Total Time: 55 minutes
218	High-Volume Endurance	Build endurance with a high-volume, low-intensity workout, focusing on maintaining a consistent stroke rate.	(1) Row for 90 minutes at a light to moderate pace.
			Total Time: 90 minutes
219	Cardiovascular & Muscular Endurance	Maintain a steady pace on the rower; focus on form and endurance during bodyweight exercises.	(1) Row for 4 minutes at moderate intensity
			Total Rounds: 4
			Time Cap: 40 minutes
220	Power Endurance	Build power endurance with high-intensity rowing intervals and strength-based bodyweight exercises.	(1) Row for 500 meters at high intensity
			Total Rounds: 3
			Time Cap: 30 minutes

Workout No.	Objective	Focus	Workout
221	Agility & Speed	Improve agility and speed with fast-paced rowing and agility-focused bodyweight exercises.	(1) Row for 2 minutes at high intensity
			Total Rounds: 5
			Time Cap: 25 minutes
222	Recovery & Technique Focus	Use rowing for active recovery while focusing on refining technique, complemented by gentle bodyweight mobility exercises.	(1) Row at a light pace for 10 minutes
			Total Rounds: 2
			Time Cap: 40 minutes
223	Enhance Cardio Efficiency	Keep your strokes consistent and focus on breathing evenly throughout the entire workout.	(1) Row at a moderate pace for 10 minutes
			(2) Rest for 2 minutes
			Repeat 3 times
			Total time: 36 minutes
224	Maximize Endurance	Aim to maintain a steady and sustainable pace, focusing on endurance rather than speed.	(1) Row for 15 minutes at a steady pace
			Total distance: Aim to increase distance with each session
225	Boost High-Intensity Power	Push yourself to the limit with each sprint; focus on maximum effort and quick recovery.	(1) 30 seconds sprint, 1 minute rest
			Total rounds: 10
226	Develop Rhythmic Consistency	Focus on maintaining a consistent stroke rate and rhythm throughout the workout.	(1) Row for 20 minutes at 22 strokes per minute
			Total distance: Measure your consistency and aim to improve

Workout No.	Objective	Focus	Workout
227	Interval Training Challenge	Alternate between high-intensity rowing and recovery periods to improve anaerobic capacity.	(1) 1 minute of high-intensity rowing, 1 minute of light rowing
			Total time: 20 minutes
228	Increase Aerobic Capacity	Maintain a moderate intensity to challenge your aerobic system without burning out.	(1) Row for 45 minutes at a moderate intensity
			Total distance: Focus on covering a greater distance each time
229	Speed and Recovery	Work on fast sprints followed by adequate recovery to improve speed and recovery time.	(1) Row 500 meters as fast as possible, 2 minutes rest
			Total rounds: 5
230	Technique and Efficiency	Concentrate on perfecting your form with each stroke to increase efficiency.	(1) Row for 30 minutes focusing on technique (catch, drive, finish, recovery)
			Total strokes: Keep count and focus on smooth, efficient movements
231	Stamina Builder	Extend your limits by maintaining a challenging pace for a longer duration.	(1) Row for 60 minutes at a consistent pace
			Total distance: Aim to maintain or slightly increase your pace throughout
232	Active Recovery Session	Use rowing as a means to recover actively, focusing on movement and light intensity.	(1) Row for 30 minutes at a light, easy pace
			Total time: Keep it relaxed focusing on recovery and enjoying the session
233	Cardiovascular Endurance	Keep your heart rate up and move quickly between rowing and exercises.	(1) Row 400m
			Total rounds: 3

Workout No.	Objective	Focus	Workout
234	Strength and Power	Focus on explosive movements during exercises and powerful strokes while rowing.	(1) Row 500m
			Total rounds: 3
235	Core Strength	Engage your core throughout the rowing and during each bodyweight exercise.	(1) Row 300m
			Total rounds: 5
236	Agility and Speed	Transition quickly between rowing and exercises to improve agility and speed.	(1) Row 200m sprint
			Total rounds: 6
237	High-Intensity Intervals	Push your limits during high-intensity rowing and recover with bodyweight movements.	(1) Row 1 min at high intensity
			Total time: 20 minutes
238	Endurance Building	Maintain a consistent, moderate pace to build endurance over time.	(1) Row 1000m
			Total rounds: 2
239	Flexibility and Recovery	Use this workout to focus on stretching and recovering muscles.	(1) Row 500m at a light pace
			Total rounds: 3
240	Balance and Coordination	Keep focused on maintaining balance during exercises and coordination during rowing.	(1) Row 300m
			Total rounds: 4

Workout No.	Objective	Focus	Workout
241	Full-Body Conditioning	Engage all muscle groups evenly throughout the workout for full-body conditioning.	(1) Row 700m
			Total rounds: 3
242	Stamina and Mental Toughness	Challenge your stamina and mental resilience by maintaining intensity throughout the workout.	(1) Row 2 km
			(2) Plank for 1 min
			Total rounds: 1, focus on completing as fast as possible
243	Cardiovascular Endurance	Focus on maintaining a steady pace to improve heart and lung health.	(1) Row for 5 minutes at moderate intensity.
			Total rounds: 6, with 1-minute rest between rounds.
244	High-Intensity Intervals	Push hard during sprints; use rest periods to recover breathing and prepare for the next burst.	(1) Row 30 seconds at maximum effort, then rest for 30 seconds.
			Total rounds: 20
245	Steady-State Training	Maintain a consistent stroke rate and intensity to build endurance.	(1) Row for 40 minutes at a consistent, moderate pace.
			Total distance: Aim for maximum meters.
246	Speed Work	Concentrate on increasing stroke rate without sacrificing form to boost speed.	(1) Row 1 minute at high stroke rate, then 1 minute at low stroke rate.
			Total time: 30 minutes
247	Anaerobic Threshold	Work at a high intensity to increase your ability to handle lactic acid build-up.	(1) Row 500 meters at high intensity, then 2 minutes rest.
			Total rounds: 5

Workout No.	Objective	Focus	Workout
248	Recovery Row	Use this gentle rowing workout to aid muscle recovery and flexibility.	(1) Row at a light intensity focusing on smooth, controlled strokes.
			Total time: 20 minutes
249	Aerobic Capacity	Build aerobic power by maintaining a challenging but sustainable intensity.	(1) Row 4 minutes at 70-75% effort, then rest 1 minute.
			Total rounds: 8
250	Technique Focus	Pay attention to rowing technique, aiming for efficiency and effectiveness in each stroke.	(1) Row 20 minutes focusing on technique; catch, drive, finish, recovery.
			Total strokes: Aim for precision and smoothness.
251	Power Strokes	Emphasize powerful, deliberate strokes to enhance strength and power output.	(1) 10 rowing strokes at maximum power, followed by 20 rowing strokes at moderate pace
			Total time: 25 minutes, alternating power and pace.
252	Interval Pyramid	Increase then decrease the length of work intervals for varied intensity.	(1) Row 1 min, rest 1 min, row 2 min, rest 1 min, up to 4 min, then back down
			Total time: Complete the pyramid cycle twice.
253	Cardio & Strength Balance	Balance effort between cardio on the rower and strength in bodyweight moves.	(1) Row 500m
			Total rounds: 3
254	High-Intensity Power	Intense row sprints paired with explosive exercises to boost power and heart rate.	(1) Row 1 min at max
			Total time: 20 minutes
255	Endurance & Core Stability	Focus on sustaining effort in rowing with core strengthening exercises.	(1) Row 1000m
			Total rounds: 2

Workout No.	Objective	Focus	Workout
256	Speed & Agility	Quick transitions between rowing sprints and agility-focused bodyweight exercises.	(1) Row 250m fast
			Total rounds: 4
257	HIIT Circuit	Alternating between rowing and high-intensity bodyweight exercises for a full-body workout.	(1) Row 2 mins hard
			Total time: Repeat for 30 mins
258	Progressive Endurance	Gradually longer rowing intervals with consistent bodyweight exercise workload.	(1) Row 500m
			(2) Row 1000m
			Total rounds: 1 of each set
259	Recovery & Mobility	Light rowing coupled with mobility-focused exercises for active recovery.	(1) Row 500m light
			Total rounds: 3
260	Full-Body Conditioning	A mix of rowing and full-body exercises to engage all muscle groups.	(1) Row 700m
			Total rounds: 3
261	Stamina Building	Long-duration rowing intervals interspersed with bodyweight exercises to build stamina.	(1) Row 2000m
			Total rounds: 1, with exercises in between
262	Core Focus Intervals	Short, intense rowing intervals with a core exercise focus between sets.	(1) Row 300m hard
			Total rounds: 4
263	Cardiovascular Fitness	Maintain a steady rhythm, focusing on breath control and consistent stroke rate.	(1) Row 30 minutes at a moderate pace.
			Total distance: Aim for a personal best in distance covered.

Workout No.	Objective	Focus	Workout
264	Interval Training	Alternate high-intensity rowing with rest periods to improve heart health and endurance.	(1) 1 min row at high intensity, 1 min rest
			Total rounds: 10
265	Endurance Building	Focus on maintaining a consistent pace, even when you start to feel tired.	(1) Row 5,000 meters at a steady pace.
			Total time: Record and aim to improve on next session.
266	Sprint Speed	Push hard during sprints; focus on quick, powerful strokes to increase your rowing speed.	(1) Row 250 meters as fast as possible, 2 mins rest
			Total rounds: 6
267	Aerobic Capacity	Keep a moderate pace that challenges you but can be maintained over time to build aerobic capacity.	(1) Row for 45 minutes at a consistent pace.
			Total distance: Aim to maximize distance covered.
268	Recovery Focus	Use light rowing to aid muscle recovery, focusing on technique and smooth movements.	(1) Row 20 minutes at a light intensity
			Total strokes: Focus on form and recovery.
269	High-Intensity Endurance	Maintain intensity over longer intervals to push your endurance and mental toughness.	(1) Row 1,000 meters at high intensity, 3 mins rest.
			Total rounds: 4
270	Technique and Efficiency	Concentrate on perfecting your rowing technique, focusing on efficient movement and form.	(1) Row 2,000 meters focusing on technique.
			Total strokes: Aim for smooth, controlled strokes.
271	Power and Strength	Execute each rowing stroke with maximum power, focusing on leg drive and arm pull-through.	(1) 10 row strokes at max power, 50 strokes at moderate pace.
			Total time: 30 minutes, alternating focus.

Workout No.	Objective	Focus	Workout
272	Progressive Intervals	Gradually increase the intensity of your rowing intervals to challenge stamina and power.	(1) Row 3 mins at 70% effort, 2 mins rest, increasing effort each round
			Total rounds: 5
273	Cardiovascular & Strength	Maintain a consistent pace on the rower and focus on form during bodyweight exercises.	(1) Row 500m
			Total rounds: 3
274	High-Intensity Intervals	Push your limits on the rower and with bodyweight exercises, with minimal rest between.	(1) Row 1 min max effort
			Total time: 20 minutes
275	Endurance & Core Strength	Keep a steady pace on the rower, and engage your core tightly during planks and leg raises.	(1) Row 1000m
			Total rounds: 2
276	Agility & Flexibility	Use the rowing sessions as active recovery and focus on fluid, dynamic movements during exercises.	(1) Row 300m
			Total rounds: 4
277	Fat Burning Circuit	Transition quickly between rowing and exercises to keep your heart rate up and maximize calorie burn.	(1) Row 2 mins
			Total rounds: As many as possible in 30 mins
278	Strength & Power	Focus on explosive power from your legs during rowing and bodyweight exercises.	(1) Row 250m sprint
			Total rounds: 4
279	Full Body Conditioning	Aim for full-body engagement and smooth transitions between rowing and exercises.	(1) Row 700m
			Total rounds: 3

Workout No.	Objective	Focus	Workout
280	Stamina Building	Maintain a challenging yet sustainable intensity to push your stamina on the rower and during exercises.	(1) Row 2000m
			(2) Row 2000m
			Total time: Aim to keep a steady pace
281	Active Recovery & Technique	Use this session for recovery, focusing on rowing technique and gentle bodyweight movements.	(1) Row 500m light
			Total rounds: 3
282	Progressive Challenge	Each round, increase the intensity on the rower and the reps for bodyweight exercises.	(1) Row 500m
			Increase rowing by 100m
			Total rounds: 4
283	Cardiovascular Health	Keep your heart rate consistently elevated; focus on steady, rhythmic breathing.	(1) Row at a moderate pace for 30 minutes.
			Total time: 30 minutes.
284	Interval Training	Push hard during the intense intervals and use the rest periods to fully recover.	(1) Row hard for 1 minute, then rest for 1 minute
			Total time: 20 minutes.
285	Endurance	Maintain a consistent, moderate effort to build stamina over a longer session.	(1) Row for 10,000 meters
			Total time: Aim for your personal best.
286	Speed Work	Focus on explosive power in each stroke during the sprints to improve speed.	(1) 250-meter sprints with 1 minute of light rowing in between.
			Total rounds: 8.

Workout No.	Objective	Focus	Workout
287	Fat Loss	Keep the intensity high with minimal rest to maximize calorie burn.	(1) 2 minutes of hard rowing followed by 1 minute of easy rowing.
			Total time: 30 minutes.
288	Aerobic Capacity	Challenge yourself to maintain a challenging but manageable pace to enhance aerobic power.	(1) Row for 45 minutes at 70% of your maximum effort
			Total distance: Record the distance.
289	High-Intensity Power	Execute each rowing stroke with maximum force; focus on quick, powerful pulls.	(1) 30 seconds of maximum effort rowing, 30 seconds rest
			Total rounds: 12.
290	Recovery	Use this workout for active recovery, focusing on technique and smooth movements.	(1) Row lightly for 20 minutes.
			Total strokes: Focus on form, not speed.
291	Technique Drill	Concentrate on perfecting your rowing technique, emphasizing efficient and effective strokes.	(1) Row at a low intensity focusing on technique for 15 minutes.
			Total time: 15 minutes.
292	Progressive Intervals	Increase intensity with each interval to challenge endurance and strength progressively.	(1) Start with rowing 500m, increase by 100m each round
			Total rounds: 5, finishing with 900m.
293	Total Body Conditioning	Focus on engaging all muscle groups evenly across rowing and exercises.	(1) Row 500m
			Total rounds: 3
294	Cardiovascular Endurance	Maintain a steady, moderate pace on the rower, keeping your heart rate up.	(1) Row 1000m
			Total rounds: 2

Workout No.	Objective	Focus	Workout
295	High-Intensity Training	Push hard during each activity, aiming for maximum effort with minimal rest.	(1) Row 1 min at max effort
			Total time: Repeat for 20 mins
296	Core & Stability Focus	Engage your core throughout the workout for stability during rowing and exercises.	(1) Row 300m
			Total rounds: 4
297	Agility & Speed	Transition quickly between rowing and bodyweight exercises to enhance agility and speed.	(1) Row 200m
			Total rounds: 5
298	Endurance & Strength	Aim for a balance between maintaining a challenging pace and performing exercises with control.	(1) Row 750m
			Total rounds: 3
299	Recovery & Mobility	Use this lighter workout to focus on rowing technique and mobility exercises.	(1) Row 400m at light intensity
			Total rounds: 3
300	Progressive Challenge	Gradually increase the rowing distance while keeping the number of bodyweight exercises consistent.	(1) Row 300m
			(2) Row 500m
			Total rounds: 1 set of each distance
301	Cardiovascular Endurance	Keep a steady pace and focus on maintaining your breathing rhythm.	(1) Row for 20 minutes at a moderate pace.
			Total time: 20 minutes.

Workout No.	Objective	Focus	Workout
302	High-Intensity Intervals	Push hard during the work intervals, then fully recover during the rests.	(1) 30 seconds rowing of all-out effort, followed by 1 minute of rest.
			Total time: Repeat for 15 minutes.
303	Endurance Building	Maintain a consistent pace, focusing on endurance rather than speed.	(1) Row for 5000 meters.
			Total distance: 5000 meters.
304	Speed Work	Concentrate on fast, powerful strokes to improve your overall rowing speed.	(1) 10 x 100 meters sprints, with 1 minute of light rowing in between.
			Total rounds: 10 sprints.
305	Fat Loss	Keep the intensity high and rest periods short to maximize calorie burn.	(1) Row 1 minute hard, 1 minute easy.
			Total time: 20 minutes.
306	Aerobic Capacity	Challenge yourself to maintain a challenging pace to improve aerobic power.	(1) Row for 40 minutes at a steady, moderate intensity.
			Total time: 40 minutes.
307	Recovery Row	Use light, steady rowing to aid recovery and focus on technique.	(1) Row for 15 minutes at a light intensity, focusing on form.
			Total time: 15 minutes.
308	Technique Focus	Pay attention to each phase of your stroke, aiming for efficiency and power.	(1) Row with focus on technique for 30 minutes.
			Total strokes: Aim for consistency and smoothness.
309	Power Strokes	Emphasize power in each stroke, focusing on leg drive and strong pull.	(1) 20 seconds of power strokes, 40 seconds of easy rowing.
			Total time: Repeat for 25 minutes.

Workout No.	Objective	Focus	Workout
310	Interval Pyramid	Increase and then decrease the length of your work intervals.	(1) Row for 1 min, rest for 1 min, row for 2 mins, rest for 1 min, continue up to 4 mins, then back down.
			Total time: Complete the pyramid.
311	Cardio & Strength Integration	Transition smoothly between rowing and bodyweight exercises to maintain heart rate and build strength.	(1) Row 500m
			Total rounds: 2
312	High-Intensity Interval Training (HIIT)	Push your maximum effort on the rower and during exercises with minimal rest for high intensity.	(1) Row 1 min at high intensity
			Total time: Repeat for 15 mins
313	Endurance & Core	Maintain endurance on the rower; focus on core stability and strength during floor exercises.	(1) Row 1000m
			Total rounds: 2
314	Power & Agility	Alternate between short, powerful rowing sprints and agility-focused bodyweight movements.	(1) Row 250m sprint
			Total rounds: 4
315	Fat Burning Circuit	Maintain a quick pace with rowing and exercises to maximize calorie burn.	(1) Row 3 mins
			Total time: 30 mins, as many rounds as possible
316	Steady-State & Strength	Focus on steady-state rowing and compound bodyweight movements for strength.	(1) Row 15 mins at a moderate pace
			Total rounds: 2
317	Interval Training	Use intervals to improve cardiovascular fitness and muscular endurance.	(1) Row 500m
			Total rounds: 3

Workout No.	Objective	Focus	Workout
318	Speed & Coordination	Enhance rowing speed and coordination with dynamic bodyweight exercises.	(1) Row 200m as fast as possible
			Total rounds: 3
319	Recovery & Mobility	Use this workout for active recovery, focusing on rowing technique and light body movements.	(1) Row 10 mins at light intensity
			Total rounds: 2
320	Progressive Challenge	Increase rowing distance each round while maintaining bodyweight exercise volume.	(1) Row 300m
			(2) Row 500m
			Total rounds: 1 cycle
321	Cardiovascular Endurance	Keep a consistent rhythm and breathing; focus on long-duration to improve heart health.	(1) Row for 60 minutes at a moderate pace
			Total distance: Aim to cover as much distance as possible.
322	High-Intensity Intervals	Alternate intense rowing bursts with recovery to boost metabolism and endurance.	(1) 1-minute row at max effort, 1-minute rest
			Total rounds: 20
323	Speed and Power	Focus on explosive strokes to increase speed and power with each interval.	(1) 10 x 100m sprints with 2 minutes rest between each sprint.
			Total distance: 1000m
324	Aerobic Capacity	Maintain a steady pace to challenge your aerobic system and increase stamina.	(1) Row for 45 minutes at 70% of your max effort.
			Total time: 45 minutes

Workout No.	Objective	Focus	Workout
325	Recovery	Use light, easy rowing to promote recovery and focus on smooth, consistent strokes.	(1) Row for 30 minutes at a light intensity.
			Total strokes: Focus on technique and relaxation.
326	Technique Drill	Concentrate on rowing technique, focusing on the catch, drive, finish, and recovery in each stroke.	(1) Row for 20 minutes, with emphasis on technique
			Total strokes: Aim for precision and efficiency.
327	Anaerobic Threshold	Push the pace to the point where it becomes difficult to breathe, enhancing anaerobic fitness.	(1) Row 500m at high intensity, 1 minute rest.
			Total rounds: 8
328	Endurance Building	Focus on maintaining a moderate effort over a prolonged period to build endurance.	(1) Row for 10,000 meters at a consistent pace
			Total time: Aim to complete in your best time possible.
329	Interval Pyramid	Increase and then decrease rowing intensity and distance to challenge endurance and strength.	(1) Row for 1, 2, 3, 4, 5 minutes with equal rest times, then back down.
			Total rounds: Complete the pyramid.
330	Stamina and Mental Toughness	Maintain focus and determination to push through longer rowing intervals at a challenging pace.	(1) Row 4 x 2000 meters with 3 minutes rest between each
			Total rounds: 4
			Total distance: 8000 meters
331	Total Body Conditioning	Engage all muscle groups through rowing and dynamic exercises for full-body conditioning.	(1) Row 500m
			Total rounds: 2

Workout No.	Objective	Focus	Workout
332	Endurance & Strength	Balance long rowing intervals with strength-building exercises for endurance and power.	(1) Row 1000m
			Total rounds: 2
333	High-Intensity Fat Burn	Alternate between high-intensity rowing and explosive exercises for maximum calorie burn.	(1) Row 2 mins hard
			Total time: 20 mins
334	Core Focus & Stability	Combine rowing with core-focused exercises for enhanced stability and abdominal strength.	(1) Row 500m
			Total rounds: 3
335	Speed & Agility	Mix quick rowing sprints with agility exercises to improve speed and coordination.	(1) Row 250m sprint
			Total rounds: 4
336	Recovery & Mobility	Utilize light rowing and gentle bodyweight movements to aid recovery and enhance mobility.	(1) Row 300m light
			Total rounds: 3
337	Interval Challenge	Push endurance with rowing intervals separated by strength exercises for a challenging workout.	(1) Row 3 mins
			Total time: 30 mins
338	Progressive Overload	Gradually increase rowing distance while maintaining consistent exercise volume for progressive training.	(1) Row 400m
			(2) Row 600m
			(3) Row 800m
			Total rounds: 1 cycle

Workout No.	Objective	Focus	Workout
339	Cardiovascular Endurance	Long-duration rowing interspersed with bodyweight exercises for sustained cardiovascular effort.	(1) Row 800m
			Total rounds: 2
340	Power & Plyometrics	Integrate rowing with plyometric exercises to enhance explosive power and muscular strength.	(1) Row 500m
			Total rounds: 3
341	Cardiovascular Endurance	Maintain a consistent pace; focus on breathing and staying in the aerobic zone for heart health.	(1) Row for 30 minutes at a moderate intensity.
			Total time: 30 minutes.
342	High-Intensity Intervals	Alternate between maximum effort and rest periods to boost cardiovascular capacity and fat burn.	(1) 40 seconds of high-intensity rowing followed by 20 seconds of rest.
			Total rounds: 15.
343	Steady-State Rowing	Focus on a sustainable pace that challenges you but can be maintained to build endurance.	(1) Row for 45 minutes at a steady pace.
			Total time: 45 minutes.
344	Speed Sprints	Push hard for short distances to improve speed and power, focusing on quick recovery during rests.	(1) 200 meters sprint, 1 minute rest
			Total rounds: 10.
345	Aerobic Threshold	Aim to row at an intensity where maintaining conversation becomes difficult, to improve aerobic fitness.	(1) Row for 2 minutes on, 1 minute off.
			Total time: 30 minutes.
346	Technique Focus	Concentrate on perfecting your stroke, paying attention to form and efficiency.	(1) 20 minutes of technique-focused rowing at a low intensity.
			Total strokes: Aim for consistent, efficient strokes.

Workout No.	Objective	Focus	Workout
347	Recovery Rowing	Use light rowing to facilitate active recovery, focusing on smooth movements.	(1) Row for 20 minutes at a light, comfortable pace.
			Total time: 20 minutes.
348	Progressive Intervals	Gradually increase the rowing intensity with each interval to build endurance and strength.	(1) Row 3 minutes easy, 2 minutes medium, 1 minute hard.
			Total rounds: 4.
349	Ladder Workout	Increase then decrease rowing distances for a challenging, pyramid-style workout.	(1) Row 250m, 500m, 750m, 1000m, 750m, 500m, 250m with 1 minute rest between each.
			Total distance: Complete the set.
350	Anaerobic Capacity	Work at high intensity to increase your body's ability to work in oxygen-debt, enhancing short burst power.	(1) 1 minute of max effort rowing, 2 minutes of rest.
			Total rounds: 8.
351	Full-Body Conditioning	Transition smoothly between rowing and exercises, maintaining high energy and focus.	(1) Row 400m
			Total rounds: 3
352	Cardiovascular Endurance	Maintain a steady, consistent pace on the rower, focusing on deep, controlled breathing.	(1) Row 1000m
			Total rounds: 2
353	High-Intensity Fat Burn	Push to your limit on the rower and with bodyweight exercises, minimizing rest times.	(1) Row 1 min all-out
			Total time: 20 mins

Workout No.	Objective	Focus	Workout
354	Strength & Endurance	Focus on powerful rowing strokes and controlled, deliberate movements in bodyweight exercises.	(1) Row 500m
			Total rounds: 3
355	Core Focus	Engage your core during rowing and concentrate on core stability during exercises.	(1) Row 300m
			Total rounds: 4
356	Speed & Agility	Work on fast, explosive rowing sessions followed by agility-focused exercises.	(1) Row 200m sprint
			Total rounds: 4
357	Recovery & Mobility	Use this lighter workout for active recovery, focusing on smooth rowing and gentle stretches.	(1) Row 500m light
			Total rounds: 3
358	Interval Challenge	Alternate between intense rowing intervals and strength-building exercises for a balanced challenge.	(1) Row 2 mins hard
			Total time: 30 mins
359	Progressive Overload	Gradually increase rowing intensity while keeping bodyweight exercises consistent for balanced improvement.	(1) Row 300m
			Total rounds: 1 set of each distance
360	Cardio & Strength Fusion	Combine moderate-intensity rowing with high-rep bodyweight exercises to enhance cardio and strength.	(1) Row 500m
			Total rounds: 3

Workout No.	Objective	Focus	Workout
361	Cardiovascular Endurance	Maintain a consistent stroke rate, focusing on endurance and efficient breathing throughout.	(1) Row for 60 minutes at a steady pace.
			Total time: 60 minutes.
362	High-Intensity Interval Training	Alternate between intense rowing bursts and short recovery periods to boost heart rate and endurance.	(1) 30 seconds of full-effort rowing, followed by 30 seconds of rest
			Total rounds: 20.
363	Speed Improvement	Focus on explosive starts and maintaining high speed over short distances to increase overall rowing speed.	(1) 10 x 100m sprints with 1 minute rest between sprints.
			Total distance: 1000m.
364	Aerobic Threshold	Row at a pace that is challenging but sustainable, aiming to improve aerobic fitness.	(1) 2 minutes on, 1 minute off, at 70-80% max effort.
			Total time: 30 minutes.
365	Recovery Rowing	Use light, smooth strokes focusing on form and recovery, allowing your muscles to relax.	(1) Row for 20 minutes at a light intensity.
			Total time: 20 minutes.
366	Anaerobic Capacity	Push beyond your comfort zone to increase your body's ability to handle intense efforts without oxygen.	(1) 1 minute of maximum effort rowing, followed by 2 minutes of rest
			Total rounds: 10.
367	Technique Focus	Concentrate on perfecting rowing technique with emphasis on the catch, drive, finish, and recovery.	(1) Row for 30 minutes, focusing on technique with every stroke.
			Total time: 30 minutes.
368	Stamina Building	Maintain a moderate, consistent pace to build stamina and resilience over longer rowing sessions.	(1) Row for 5000m.
			Total distance: 5000m.

Workout No.	Objective	Focus	Workout
369	Interval Pyramid	Gradually increase the length of work intervals before decreasing, challenging both endurance and intensity.	(1) Row for 1, 2, 3, 4, 5 minutes with 1 minute rest between intervals, then back down.
			Total time: Complete the pyramid.
370	Power and Endurance	Blend short, high-power bursts with longer, moderate-intensity intervals to enhance both power and endurance.	(1) Row 250m at high power, then row 1000m at moderate pace. Repeat
			Total rounds: 4.
			Total distance: Aim for strong, powerful strokes during the 250m sprints.
371	Cardio & Strength Integration	Balance the cardiovascular effort on the rower with strength-building bodyweight exercises.	(1) Row 400m
			Total rounds: 3
372	Endurance & Core Strength	Maintain endurance on the rower; focus on core strength during bodyweight exercises.	(1) Row 800m
			Total rounds: 2
373	High-Intensity Fat Burn	Maximize calorie burn with high-intensity rowing intervals and quick bodyweight movements.	(1) Row 2 mins at high intensity
			Total time: 20 mins
374	Strength & Agility	Focus on building strength with bodyweight exercises and improving agility with rowing.	(1) Row 300m
			Total rounds: 4
375	Recovery & Mobility	Use rowing as active recovery and bodyweight exercises to enhance mobility.	(1) Row 500m light
			Total rounds: 3

Workout No.	Objective	Focus	Workout
376	Interval Challenge	Push endurance with challenging rowing intervals and strengthening bodyweight exercises.	(1) Row 3 mins
			Total time: 30 mins
377	Progressive Overload	Increase rowing intensity while maintaining consistent volume in bodyweight exercises for overall growth.	(1) Row 300m
			(2) Row 400m
			(3) Row 500m
			Total rounds: 1 set of each distance
378	Speed & Power	Combine short, powerful rowing sprints with explosive bodyweight exercises for speed and power.	(1) Row 250m sprint
			Total rounds: 3
379	Full-Body Conditioning	Engage all major muscle groups through rowing and comprehensive bodyweight exercises.	(1) Row 500m
			Total rounds: 2
380	Cardiovascular Endurance	Maintain a consistent pace to enhance heart and lung function, focusing on endurance over speed.	(1) Row for 45 minutes at a moderate intensity.
			Total time: 45 minutes.
381	High-Intensity Intervals	Alternate intense rowing with rest periods to boost cardiovascular and muscular endurance.	(1) 1 min row at max effort, 1 min rest.
			Total rounds: 15.
382	Speed Development	Work on increasing stroke rate for short bursts to improve overall rowing speed.	(1) 8 x 250m sprints with 2 mins rest between each
			Total distance: 2000m.

Workout No.	Objective	Focus	Workout
383	Aerobic Power	Row at a challenging but sustainable pace to build aerobic capacity and stamina.	(1) Row for 2 mins at 80% effort, 1 min easy row.
			Total time: 30 mins.
384	Recovery Focus	Use gentle rowing to facilitate muscle recovery and improve flexibility, focusing on smooth and controlled movements.	(1) Row for 20 minutes at a light intensity, focusing on form.
			Total time: 20 minutes.
385	Technique and Efficiency	Concentrate on rowing technique, emphasizing posture, stroke consistency, and efficiency.	(1) Row with focus on technique for 30 minutes at a low intensity
			Total strokes: Aim for consistency and smoothness.
386	Endurance Building	Maintain a moderate intensity over an extended period to increase endurance without overexerting.	(1) Row for 10,000 meters
			Total distance: 10,000m
387	Interval Pyramid	Gradually increase and then decrease the intensity and length of intervals to challenge endurance and mental toughness.	(1) Row 1, 2, 3, 4, 5 mins with 2 mins rest between, then back down.
			Total time: Complete the full pyramid.
388	Stamina and Mental Resilience	Keep a steady pace in longer rowing sessions to build physical stamina and mental resilience.	(1) 3 x 2000m with 3 mins rest between sets
			Total distance: 6000m.
389	Power Stroke Focus	Enhance power output with each stroke, focusing on leg drive and arm pull-through.	(1) 20 seconds of power strokes, 40 seconds of easy rowing for recovery
			Total time: 20 minutes, alternating power and recovery.
390	Full-Body Conditioning	Engage all major muscle groups evenly for balanced strength and endurance.	(1) Row 500m
			Total rounds: 3

Workout No.	Objective	Focus	Workout
398	Agility and Coordination	Focus on quick transitions and maintaining agility throughout the workout.	(1) Row 250m
			Total rounds: 3
399	Stamina and Resilience	Build stamina and mental resilience with longer rowing intervals and consistent exercises.	(1) Row 800m
			Total rounds: 2
400	Cardiovascular Endurance	Maintain a consistent pace, focusing on your breathing and endurance.	(1) Row for 30 minutes at a moderate, steady pace.
			Total time: 30 minutes.
401	High-Intensity Intervals	Alternate intense rowing bursts with rest periods for maximum calorie burn.	(1) 1 min max effort row, 1 min rest.
			Total rounds: 10.
402	Speed Development	Concentrate on increasing stroke rate for short distances to boost speed.	(1) 8 x 200m sprints, 2 mins rest between sprints.
			Total distance: 1600m.
403	Aerobic Threshold Training	Aim to row at a pace where it's challenging but sustainable for aerobic gains.	(1) 4 x 5 min row at 80% effort, 3 mins rest between intervals.
			Total time: 32 minutes.
404	Recovery Focus	Use light rowing to facilitate active recovery, focusing on smooth strokes.	(1) Row for 20 minutes at a light intensity, emphasizing form.
			Total time: 20 minutes.
405	Technique and Efficiency	Dedicate time to refining stroke technique, ensuring efficient movement throughout.	(1) 30 minutes of technique-focused rowing at a low intensity.
			Total strokes: Aim for consistency.

Workout No.	Objective	Focus	Workout
406	Endurance Building	Engage in longer rowing sessions to improve stamina and endurance capacity.	(1) Row for 5000m.
			Total distance: 5000m, aim for personal best time.
407	Interval Pyramid	Gradually increase and then decrease the effort and duration of rowing intervals.	(1) Row 1, 2, 3, 4, 5 minutes, then back down, with 2 mins rest between
			Total time: Complete the pyramid.
408	Power Stroke Work	Emphasize the power and strength in each stroke for short intervals.	(1) 20 secs of power strokes, 40 secs easy rowing for recovery.
			Total time: 20 minutes.
409	Mental Toughness Challenge	Push through longer distances to build resilience and mental fortitude.	(1) 2 x 2000m row with 5 mins rest between sets.e.
			Total distance: 4000m, focus on maintaining pac
410	Full-Body Blast	Engage your entire body, alternating between rowing and dynamic exercises for full-body conditioning.	(1) Row 500m
			Total rounds: 2
411	Cardio Endurance	Maintain a steady pace on the rower, focusing on endurance and consistency in exercises.	(1) Row 1000m
			Total rounds: 2
412	HIIT Challenge	Maximize effort with intense rowing and bodyweight exercises, keeping rest to a minimum.	(1) Row 1 min at max effort
			Total time: 20 mins
413	Core & Stability	Strengthen core muscles and improve stability through focused rowing and core exercises.	(1) Row 400m
			Total rounds: 3

Workout No.	Objective	Focus	Workout
414	Power & Speed	Develop power and speed with short rowing sprints and explosive bodyweight movements.	(1) Row 200m sprint
			Total rounds: 4
415	Active Recovery	Focus on recovery with light rowing and gentle bodyweight exercises to enhance mobility.	(1) Row 300m light
			Total rounds: 3
416	Endurance & Strength	Build endurance with longer rowing intervals and strength with high-rep bodyweight exercises.	(1) Row 750m
			Total rounds: 2
417	Interval Mix	Challenge both aerobic and anaerobic systems with mixed intervals and bodyweight resistance.	(1) Row 3 mins hard
			Total time: 30 mins
418	Agility & Coordination	Enhance agility and coordination with quick rowing intervals and agility-focused exercises.	(1) Row 250m
			Total rounds: 3
419	Stamina Builder	Increase stamina with extended rowing sessions and maintain intensity in bodyweight exercises.	(1) Row 800m
			Total rounds: 2
420	Cardiovascular Fitness	Maintain a consistent pace to build endurance, focusing on staying in the aerobic zone.	(1) Row for 40 minutes at a moderate pace.
			Total time: 40 minutes.
421	High-Intensity Intervals	Alternate between high-intensity rowing and rest periods to increase heart rate and improve endurance.	(1) 30 seconds max effort rowing, 30 seconds rest.
			Total rounds: 20.

Workout No.	Objective	Focus	Workout
422	Endurance & Stamina	Keep a steady pace, focusing on building stamina and maintaining endurance throughout the session.	(1) Row for 60 minutes at a steady pace.
			Total time: 60 minutes.
423	Speed & Agility	Work on short, high-speed bursts to improve rowing agility and speed.	(1) 15 x 200m sprints with 1 minute rest between each.
			Total distance: 3000m.
424	Aerobic Power	Row at a challenging but manageable pace to increase aerobic capacity.	(1) 5 x 4 minutes at 75% effort, with 2 minutes rest between intervals.
			Total time: 30 minutes.
425	Recovery & Technique	Use light rowing to focus on recovery and technique improvement, paying attention to form.	(1) Row for 20 minutes at a light intensity, focusing on stroke technique.
			Total time: 20 minutes.
426	Threshold Training	Push yourself just below the anaerobic threshold to improve your rowing efficiency at high intensities.	(1) 4 x 1000m with 3 minutes rest between, aiming to keep a consistent pace that feels challenging but sustainable.
			Total distance: 4000m.
427	Interval Pyramid	Increase intensity with pyramid intervals, focusing on both endurance and power.	(1) Row 1, 2, 3, 4, 5 minutes with equal time rest between, then reverse back down.
			Total time: Complete the pyramid sequence.
428	Mental Toughness	Maintain focus and perseverance through longer, challenging rowing intervals.	(1) 2 x 2000m row with 5 minutes rest between. Aim to maintain or improve time on the second 2000m
			Total distance: 4000m.
429	Dynamic Warm-up & Cooldown	Incorporate a dynamic warm-up followed by a focused rowing session and a comprehensive cooldown.	(1) Row 5 minutes light, then 10 x 1 minute at moderate intensity with 1 minute easy rowing for recovery, followed by 5 minutes
			Total time: 25 minutes.

Workout No.	Objective	Focus	Workout
430	Total Body Conditioning	Engage your whole body through a mix of rowing and dynamic bodyweight movements for strength and endurance.	(1) Row 500m Total rounds: 3
431	Cardiovascular & Core Strength	Balance cardiovascular rowing sessions with core-strengthening exercises to enhance endurance and core stability.	(1) Row 1000m Total rounds: 2
432	High-Intensity Fat Burn	Combine high-intensity rowing intervals with bodyweight exercises to maximize calorie burn and improve cardiovascular health.	(1) Row 2 mins hard Total time: 20 mins
433	Strength & Agility	Integrate rowing sprints with agility-focused bodyweight exercises to build strength and improve agility.	(1) Row 300m fast Total rounds: 4
434	Endurance & Mobility	Use longer rowing distances to build endurance, paired with mobility exercises for full-body flexibility.	(1) Row 750m Total rounds: 3
435	Power Interval Training	Focus on powerful, explosive rowing intervals followed by high-intensity bodyweight exercises for power development.	(1) Row 250m sprint Total rounds: 4
436	Active Recovery	Incorporate light rowing with gentle bodyweight movements to aid recovery and enhance mobility.	(1) Row 400m light Total rounds: 3

Workout No.	Objective	Focus	Workout
437	Progressive Challenge	Gradually increase rowing intensity while maintaining consistent exercise volume for a progressive challenge.	(1) Row 300m
			(2) 20 Sit-ups
			(3) Row 400m
			Total rounds: 1 set of each distance
438	Cardio & Core Blast	Mix moderate-intensity rowing with core-focused exercises for a cardio and abdominal strength workout.	(1) Row 500m
			Total rounds: 3
439	Speed & Endurance Circuit	Enhance speed with short rowing sprints and build endurance with compound bodyweight exercises.	(1) Row 200m as fast as possible
			Total rounds: 3
440	Cardiovascular Endurance	Keep a consistent rhythm, focusing on maintaining a steady pace to build endurance.	(1) Row for 30 minutes at a moderate intensity.
			Total time: 30 minutes.
441	High-Intensity Intervals	Push hard during intense intervals and focus on recovery during rest periods to enhance cardiovascular health.	(1) 1 min of high-intensity rowing followed by 1 min of rest.
			Total rounds: 15.
442	Speed Boost	Work on increasing your stroke rate and power during short bursts to improve speed.	(1) 20 x 100m sprints with 45 seconds rest between sprints.
			Total distance: 2000m.
443	Endurance Building	Maintain a moderate, consistent pace, focusing on long-duration endurance.	(1) Row for 10,000 meters
			Total distance: 10,000m.

Workout No.	Objective	Focus	Workout
444	Aerobic Threshold	Row at a pace that is challenging but sustainable, aiming to push your aerobic threshold.	(1) 4 x 5 minutes at 80% effort, 3 minutes rest between intervals. Total time: 32 minutes.
445	Interval Pyramid	Gradually increase the length and intensity of your intervals for a challenging and varied workout.	(1) Row for 1, 2, 3, 4, 5 minutes with equal rest times, then back down. Total time: Complete the set.
446	Stamina and Mental Toughness	Focus on maintaining a challenging pace in longer intervals to build stamina and resilience.	(1) 3 x 2000m with 4 minutes rest between each set Total distance: 6000m.
447	Power and Strength	Emphasize powerful strokes to maximize force output and build rowing strength.	(1) 10 x 30 seconds of maximum effort rowing, 1 minute rest between. Total rounds: 10.
448	Dynamic Warm-up and Cooldown	Start with a dynamic warm-up on the rower, followed by a structured workout, and end with a cooldown.	(1) Row 5 minutes at a light pace to warm up, then row 10 x 2 minutes at moderate intensity with 1 minute rest, followed by 5 Total time: 35 minutes.
449	Full-Body Conditioning	Engage your entire body by alternating between rowing and dynamic bodyweight exercises for a comprehensive workout.	(1) Row 500m Total rounds: 3
450	Cardiovascular Endurance	Maintain a steady heart rate with consistent pacing on the rower, interspersed with bodyweight exercises to build endurance.	(1) Row 1000m Total rounds: 2

Workout No.	Objective	Focus	Workout
451	High-Intensity Fat Burn	Alternate between high-intensity rowing intervals and explosive bodyweight movements to maximize calorie burn and cardiovascular benefits.	(1) Row 2 mins at high intensity
			Total time: 20 mins
452	Strength & Agility	Pair rowing sprints with agility-focused bodyweight exercises to enhance muscular strength and improve agility.	(1) Row 300m fast
			Total rounds: 4
453	Endurance & Mobility	Build endurance with longer rowing intervals and incorporate mobility exercises to improve flexibility and reduce injury risk.	(1) Row 750m
			Total rounds: 3
454	Power Interval Training	Focus on powerful, explosive rowing intervals combined with high-intensity bodyweight exercises to build power and endurance.	(1) Row 250m sprint
			Total rounds: 4
455	Active Recovery	Use light rowing and gentle bodyweight exercises to promote recovery while maintaining movement and flexibility.	(1) Row 400m light
			Total rounds: 3
456	Progressive Challenge	Gradually increase rowing intensity and maintain consistency in bodyweight exercise volume to challenge stamina and strength progressively.	(1) Row 300m
			(2) Row 400m
			(3) Row 500m
			Total rounds: 1 set of each distance

Workout No.	Objective	Focus	Workout
457	Cardio & Core Blast	Combine moderate-intensity rowing intervals with core-strengthening exercises for a balanced cardio and abdominal workout.	(1) Row 500m
			Total rounds: 3
458	Speed & Endurance Circuit	Enhance speed with quick rowing intervals and build endurance with sustained, compound bodyweight movements.	(1) Row 200m as fast as possible
			Total rounds: 3
459	Cardiovascular Endurance	Maintain a consistent stroke rate and focus on your breathing to enhance endurance and stamina.	(1) Row for 45 minutes at a steady pace.
			Total time: 45 minutes.
460	High-Intensity Intervals	Push your limits with intense rowing bursts followed by brief recovery periods to improve cardiovascular health.	(1) 20 seconds of all-out rowing, followed by 40 seconds of rest.
			Total rounds: 20.
461	Speed Improvement	Concentrate on fast, powerful strokes to increase your rowing speed over short distances.	(1) 12 x 250m sprints with 1 minute of rest between each sprint.
			Total distance: 3000m.
462	Endurance Building	Aim for a moderate, consistent pace that you can maintain over a longer period to build endurance.	(1) Row for 10,000 meters at a moderate pace.
			Total distance: 10,000m.
463	Aerobic Power	Row at a challenging pace to increase your aerobic capacity without hitting the anaerobic zone.	(1) 5 x 1000m with 3 minutes rest between sets at 75% of your max effort
			Total rounds: 5.
464	Recovery Focus	Use the rower for a low-intensity session focusing on technique and recovery.	(1) Row for 20 minutes at a light intensity, focusing on perfecting your stroke.
			Total time: 20 minutes.

Workout No.	Objective	Focus	Workout
465	Interval Pyramid	Challenge yourself with intervals that increase then decrease in length to test both your endurance and speed.	(1) Row for 1, 2, 3, 4, 5 minutes, rest for the same duration between intervals, then reverse.
			Total time: Complete the pyramid sequence.
466	Stamina & Mental Toughness	Develop your stamina and mental fortitude with a long, challenging rowing session.	(1) 2 x 5000m with 5 minutes rest between each piece
			Total distance: 10,000m.
467	Power Training	Focus on maximizing the power of each stroke, with an emphasis on leg drive and strong pulls.	(1) 30 seconds of maximum effort rowing, 1 minute of easy rowing for recovery
			Total time: 20 minutes, alternating between power and recovery.
468	Dynamic Warm-Up & Cool Down	Start and end your workout with a rowing session that gradually increases then decreases in intensity.	(1) Row 5 minutes increasing intensity every minute, perform main workout (choose any above), then row 5 minutes decreasing
			Total time: Varies with main workout.
469	Total Body Conditioning	Engage every major muscle group for balanced strength and endurance through rowing and comprehensive body movements.	(1) Row 500m
			Total rounds: 2
470	Cardiovascular Endurance	Maintain a steady pace on the rower to build endurance, interspersed with exercises to keep your heart rate up.	(1) Row 1000m
			Total rounds: 2
471	High-Intensity Fat Burn	Alternate between high-intensity rowing and quick bodyweight exercises for maximum calorie burn.	(1) Row 2 mins at high intensity
			Total time: 20 mins
472	Strength & Power	Focus on explosive power with short rowing sprints and strength-building bodyweight exercises.	(1) Row 200m sprint
			Total rounds: 4

Workout No.	Objective	Focus	Workout
473	Endurance & Stability	Combine longer rowing intervals with stability-focused bodyweight exercises to enhance endurance and core stability.	(1) Row 750m
			Total rounds: 3
474	Recovery & Flexibility	Use light rowing and bodyweight stretching exercises to promote recovery and flexibility.	(1) Row 500m light
			Total rounds: 3
475	Aerobic Threshold Push	Challenge your aerobic threshold with rowing intervals followed by bodyweight exercises to keep intensity high.	(1) Row 3 mins hard
			Total time: 30 mins
476	Interval Challenge	Test both your aerobic and anaerobic systems with a mix of rowing and high-intensity bodyweight intervals.	(1) Row 1 min all-out
			Total rounds: 8
477	Speed & Agility Focus	Improve your rowing speed and overall agility with fast-paced rowing and agility drills.	(1) Row 250m as fast as possible
			Total rounds: 4
478	Stamina & Resilience Building	Build long-term stamina and resilience with a prolonged, challenging workout combining rowing and endurance exercises.	(1) Row 800m
			Total rounds: 2
479	Cardiovascular Health	Maintain a steady, moderate pace to enhance heart health without overexertion.	(1) Row for 30 minutes at a consistent, moderate pace.
			Total time: 30 minutes.
480	High-Intensity Training	Alternate between high-intensity rowing and rest to boost metabolism and endurance.	(1) 1 minute of intense rowing, followed by 1 minute of rest.
			Total rounds: 15.

Workout No.	Objective	Focus	Workout
481	Speed Development	Focus on short, fast bursts to increase your rowing speed and explosive power.	(1) 10 x 100m sprints with 1 minute rest between each.
			Total distance: 1000m.
482	Endurance Building	Aim for a longer, continuous rowing session at a moderate pace to build stamina.	(1) Row for 60 minutes at a steady pace.
			Total time: 60 minutes.
483	Aerobic Capacity	Enhance aerobic fitness by maintaining a challenging yet sustainable pace.	(1) 5 x 4 minutes at 70-75% max effort, with 2 minutes rest between sets.
			Total time: 30 minutes.
484	Recovery Row	Utilize a low-intensity rowing session to aid in muscle recovery and flexibility.	(1) Row gently for 20 minutes focusing on form and recovery.
			Total time: 20 minutes.
485	Anaerobic Threshold	Push just beyond comfort to improve high-intensity endurance and power.	(1) 4 x 500m with 3 minutes rest, aiming for high intensity.
			Total rounds: 4.
486	Interval Pyramid	Increase and then decrease the intensity and duration of rowing intervals.	(1) Row for 1, 2, 3, 4, 5, 4, 3, 2, 1 minutes with 1 minute rest between each.
			Total time: Approx. 36 minutes.
487	Stamina & Resilience	Extend your capacity for prolonged effort with a challenging distance row.	(1) Row a single 10k as fast as possible.
			Total distance: 10,000m.
488	Dynamic Warm-Up & Cooldown	Begin with a gradual warm-up, followed by structured rowing, ending in a cooldown.	(1) Start with 5 minutes easy rowing, then 20 minutes at a moderate pace, finishing with 5 minutes cooling down.
			Total time: 30 minutes.

Workout No.	Objective	Focus	Workout
489	Comprehensive Conditioning	Engage your whole body by combining rowing with exercises for strength and endurance.	(1) Row 500m
			Total rounds: 3
490	Cardiovascular Endurance	Keep a consistent rhythm on the rower, adding exercises to challenge your heart further.	(1) Row 1000m
			Total rounds: 2
491	High-Intensity Burn	Maximize calorie burn with intense rowing and high-speed bodyweight exercises.	(1) Row 1 min hard
			Total time: 15 mins
492	Power & Strength	Focus on power during short rowing intervals and strength with bodyweight exercises.	(1) Row 250m sprint
			Total rounds: 4
493	Core & Stability	Strengthen core and improve stability with rowing and targeted bodyweight movements.	(1) Row 500m
			Total rounds: 3
494	Recovery & Mobility	Use low-intensity rowing and dynamic stretching exercises for recovery and flexibility.	(1) Row 400m gentle
			Total rounds: 3
495	Aerobic Threshold Training	Challenge your aerobic capacity with rowing and maintain intensity with bodyweight exercises.	(1) Row 4 mins moderate
			Total time: 30 mins
496	Interval & Endurance Mix	Test endurance with mixed intervals of rowing and bodyweight exercises for resilience.	(1) Row 2 mins hard
			Total rounds: 6

Workout No.	Objective	Focus	Workout
497	Speed & Agility	Enhance speed with fast-paced rowing and agility exercises.	(1) Row 200m fast
			Total rounds: 4
498	Stamina Building	Build long-term stamina with prolonged rowing and consistent bodyweight exercises.	(1) Row 800m
			Total rounds: 2
499	Cardiovascular Endurance	Focus on maintaining a steady pace, improving heart health, and increasing stamina.	(1) Row for 5,000 meters at a moderate pace.
			Total distance: 5,000 meters.
500	High-Intensity Intervals	Alternate intense rowing bursts with short recovery periods to enhance cardiovascular fitness and fat burn.	(1) 30 seconds of intense rowing, followed by 30 seconds of rest.
			Total time: 20 minutes.

<u>Dear valued customer,</u>

We are a small family-owned business, and we'd like to please kindly ask you to leave us a review.

We don't have the same budget as big publishing companies, so your support would be really appreciated. Your feedback will mean a lot to us, and we thank you in advance!

To leave your review, please scan this QR code:

Mauricio & Devon

FREE DOWNLOAD

BONUS No 1

Get the LOGGING SHEETS for free! Just scan the following QR code.

You can download them to your computer or laptop.

Print as many copies as you need to keep track of your workouts, or you can even fill them out on your device.

www.ingramcontent.com/pod-product-compliance
Lightning Source LLC
Chambersburg PA
CBHW050219270326
41914CB00003BA/476